A Paralyzing Fear

The Triumph Over Polio
in America

A Paralyzing Fear

The Triumph Over Polio in America

Nina Gilden Seavey
Jane S. Smith
Paul Wagner

TV Books
New York

Seavey, Nina Gilden.
    A paralyzing fear: the triumph over polio in America/
    by Nina Gilden Seavey, Jane S. Smith, and Paul Wagner.-
    1st ed.
        p.cm.
        Companion volume to the film: A paralyzing fear, directed
    by Nina Gilden Seavey.
        ISBN: 1-57500-070-9
        1. Poliomyelitis—United States—History. 2.
    Poliomyelitis—Vaccination—History. 3. Poliomyelitis
    vaccine—History. 4. March of Dimes Birth Defects
    Foundation—History. I. Smith, Jane S. II. Wagner, Paul,
    1948-III. Title.

    RA644.P9S43 1998   614.5'49'0973
                                        QBI98-943

"A Paralyzing Fear" was supported by:
The National Endowment for the Humanities
The Corporation for Public Broadcasting
Wyeth-Ayerst Laboratories
The George Washington University

TV Books, L.L.C.
Publishers serving the television industry.
1619 Broadway, Ninth floor
New York, NY 10019

Editorial services supplied by Rick Firstman
Text and jacket design by Joe Gannon
Manufactured in the United States

This book is dedicated to the nearly 600,000 Americans alive today who survived their bout with polio and the thousands more who died too soon

and to the memory of Dr. Jonas Salk and Dr. Albert Sabin who developed the vaccines that may soon rid the earth of this dread disease.

Authors' Note

The interviews contained in this volume were conducted with the intent of being used in the film *A Paralyzing Fear: The Story of Polio in America,* for which this book is a companion. As they are presented in the book, we have frequently edited these interviews to make them more readable as a coherent narrative. We have not, however, in any instance changed the context, tone, or substance of the original interviews.

Further, the archival photographs found throughout this book are to be interpreted as illustrations for the text. They are intended to create an ambiance for the reader of what life was like during the years of trial and then conquest over polio. These images are representative of the text and should not be construed as exact evidence or artifacts of events depicted within the text.

Specifically, within the Voices interview sections, the historical images selected within the body of the text are not personal photos of the individuals, but rather are illustrative of the experiences described in the interviews. The photograph that introduces each interview is a contemporary image of each interviewee, captured from the footage we shot on location while in production on the film.

In an effort to maintain a narrative flow and to create a presentation of the images reminiscent of a scrapbook of the polio years, we have placed the description of each image in the back of the volume beginning on page 281 in the section entitled "Catalog of Archival Photographs." This presentation has allowed us to elaborate on each image with additional insights as well as to provide the requisite photo credit. By ordering the historical essays, the interviews, the photos, and the description of illustrations in this way, we have tried to create a seamless journey through the years of pain, hope, and triumph that is the amazing story of polio in America.

Contents

Preface

Seldom in history has a society completed the full cycle of disease—from illness to epidemic to cure. Polio is America's most notable exception. It came and went in the first half of the twentieth century, and the nation was indelibly transformed by its presence. Those long polio summers tested the American people's will to live, to transcend pain and fear, and to forge their energies in the conquest of a cruel virus. Now, living under the specter of AIDS and other new viral diseases, it is important for us to understand the way in which epidemic disease fundamentally changes who we are as a people and how we coalesce to combat an unseen enemy.

The story of polio is many stories. It is a story of individuals—the terrifying onset of the symptoms in their bodies, the bewildering and wholly unanticipated chapter of their life that follows, and the intense testing of courage as each of them struggles to regain the health they so suddenly lost. It is a story about the isolation of these victims of disease, the shunning of their families, and the trepidations of those who never contract the disease but live in fear of it. And it is a story about the collective commitment demanded on all fronts—medical, scientific, political, and social—in order to conquer epidemic disease. It is the story of America's triumph over polio.

This book, and the film also entitled *A Paralyzing Fear* that it accompanies, are the result of four years of research and creative development. The project originated in the summer of 1994 at the Institute for Historical Documentary Filmmaking of the George Washington University. There, in an academic setting in which ideas could be fully developed and with the collaboration of an insightful group of students, it became clear that no serious work on the culture of epidemic disease, and specifically America's experience of polio, had ever been rendered on film. There had been documentary treatments of Salk and Sabin's horse race to discover a vaccine, but never had polio's impact on American society and culture been explored.

To help us tell this important story, we gathered a distinguished panel of advisors—historians of medicine, anthropologists, physicians specializing in polio, and popular writers on the subject. Among them was the central actor in the great drama of polio in America—Jonas Salk. Unfortunately, Dr. Salk died four days before our first taped interview with him was scheduled to begin. But throughout the creation of the film, we have been guided and inspired by his exhortation that "finally, there will be a film about what polio really meant and why it so profoundly changed this nation!"

The archival nature of the film and this book led us to conduct extensive research in repositories throughout America. But the vast majority of our material came from the March of Dimes Birth Defects Foundation. Their archive of three thousand films and five thousand photographs had never been seen before by the American public. By 1962 polio was conquered and the March of Dimes changed its focus away from this disease and began a new chapter in its history as the leader in the fight against birth defects. The large repository of images taken by this national grass-roots organization throughout the 1940s and 1950s was boxed and put into storage in a warehouse in Fort Lee, New Jersey. It stayed there—untouched by archivists, historians, writers, or filmmakers—until September of 1996 when the March of Dimes generously opened this treasure trove to us.

In these boxes we discovered a sweeping portrait of America at mid-century attempting to combat an unseen enemy. Included in the collection were rare films of President Franklin Delano Roosevelt at his second home in Warm Springs—not the FDR of the newsreels, disguising the fact of his disability in order to project an image of presidential strength, but Roosevelt the paraplegic, at home with his fellow "polios" and not at all self-conscious about his disability. Secreted in the vast repository were depictions of the vaccine research, patient treatment, and training for nurses and doctors supported by the March of Dimes. But most vivid of all were the images suggesting how this organization came to define the modern, grass-roots charity—the movie star spokesperson, the "poster child," the "Mother's March"—which mobilized average citizens in the fight against disease.

But these archival images and the history they illustrate represented only one layer of our story. There was a deeper, more human dimension left to be explored.

And so we traveled across America talking to polio victims, their families, doctors, nurses, scientists, and everyday people whose lives where indelibly altered by the annual epidemics—over forty interviews on film and another sixty on audiotape. Perhaps the most remarkable thing we discovered was that most people who had polio had largely repressed the memories of their early experiences with the disease. In today's culture, "support groups" and notions of "empowerment" set the agenda for victims of disease. But in the 1950s, the challenge for thousands of children and young adults crippled by polio was not to complain but to conform to the mainstream—to compensate for their disabilities by "pulling themselves up by the bootstraps" and moving on with their lives, no matter how different, or difficult, that life had become.

As we traveled the country interviewing the polio population, it was as if we were opening a box that had been closed for decades. Because these individuals had never talked about the toll the disease had taken on them and on their families, they often struggled to express their pain, both the pain of the disease itself and the psychological pain associated with an experience that radically altered their vision of themselves and their relationships with family and friends. Many tears were shed during our interview sessions. But no one backed away from the hard memories of the polio years.

Thus did the overarching theme of memory—how we remember our childhoods and how we reconstruct history in the collective memory—become central to our enterprise. We concluded that the film and this book must blend a broad historical account of the history of polio in America with the intensely personal memories of those who lived it. Only in this way could we re-create for today's viewer and reader those haunting summers when a virus came and terrorized a nation.

Apart from our creative aspirations for the project, there is also a social purpose we hope to achieve through this work. Over the past decade, many parents have come to question the need for vaccination for their children. According to the Centers for Disease Control and

Prevention, one in five children are not up-to-date on their immunizations by age two. In some places in America, nine out of ten babies are not current with their immunizations. While most children must be immunized prior to entrance to kindergarten, a failure to adhere to the vaccination schedule, which begins at birth and continues consistently throughout the early childhood years, clearly puts young children at extreme risk at a vulnerable time in life. So our work is particularly meant for today's parents, those too young to remember the terror that gripped America every summer and stole the life and limbs of tens of thousands of children.

Further, we must not persuade ourselves that just because polio has been conquered in this hemisphere doesn't mean it is no longer a problem throughout the rest of the world. In Africa and Asia, in crowded slums and in remote villages where vaccine arrives on camelback, there is much left to be accomplished. Leading the movement are Rotary International, the World Health Organization, the Centers for Disease Control, UNICEF, and USAID. But this exacting work must have the American public's recognition and support.

Although the film and book fundamentally comprise a history of the war against polio, we felt it was important to document these contemporary battles. In India we witnessed the Indian National Immunization Day in which 127 million children were inoculated against the disease in a single day. We also filmed the treatment of polio-afflicted children in the only hospital in the slums of Delhi. There, we came upon a father holding a two-year-old child whose leg had been seriously affected by polio. A medical technician was pouring hot wax on this child's leg, and he was screaming. Such a treatment has not been used in America since the early part of this century. While shooting this scene, cinematographer Reuben Aaronson never wavered. But when he finally lowered the eyepiece of the camera, tears were streaming down his face. We all shared his anguish at the sight of a cruel and pointless treatment for a disease that should have been eradicated long ago. This is but one of the many experiences during the year and a half of production that gave our work a deeper sense of purpose.

Over the course of creating A *Paralyzing Fear*, many persons and organizations have given of their time and energy to make the film and book a reality.

First and foremost are the scores of individuals whose lives were touched by polio when they were young, who survived, and who have brought their stories to us here. They speak for the 600,000 others who contracted the disease and are still alive today. It is their willingness to delve into difficult memories—lying helpless in an iron lung, the pain of an arched spine in the acute phase of the disease, the arduous years of rehabilitation—that has given our story its heart.

Throughout the conceptualization and execution of the project, we have enjoyed the guidance of an expert board of advisors, including Edward Berkowitz, Ph.D., Hugh Gallagher, Lauro Halstead, M.D., Alan Kraut, Ph.D., Naomi Naierman, Naomi Rogers, Ph.D., Jessica Scheer, Ph.D., Jane Smith, Ph.D., and Daniel Wilson, Ph.D. We have been thoughtfully assisted on the film by our senior production advisors Ward Chamberlin, Henry Hampton, and Geoffrey Ward. We are indebted to The George Washington University for supporting this project from its very first glimmer of an idea until now.

In addition to the substantial contribution by the March of Dimes of their archive, we tapped many other repositories in the course of producing both the film and this volume. They include: The Bettmann Archives, Cincinnati Medical Heritage Center, Hauck Center for the Albert B. Sabin Archives, the Library of Congress, the Minnesota Historical Society, the Museum of the City of New York, the National Archives, the New York Municipal Archive, the New York Public Library, *The New York Times*, the Rancho Los Amigos Medical Center, the Roosevelt Warm Springs Institute for Rehabilitation, the Franklin D. Roosevelt Library in Hyde Park, Rotary International, the Sabin Foundation, the Jonas Salk Trust, the Tuskegee University, the University of San Diego, the University of South Carolina and the D.T. Watson Rehabilitation Services.

We are tremendously grateful to the National Endowment for the Humanities, the Corporation for Public Broadcasting, and our corporate underwriter, Wyeth-Ayerst Laboratories, for providing financial support for the production and presentation of the film, and to Oregon Public Broadcasting and PBS for supporting the broadcast of the film. Wyeth Lederle Vaccines' commitment to the film's public education campaign has focused national attention on one of this project's central messages—the importance of immunization for all children.

Further, we owe a debt of gratitude to our coauthor of this book, Jane S. Smith, who also wrote *Patenting the Sun: Polio and the Salk Vaccine*. Her fluent and vivid prose renders the story so well in this book and served as the basis for much of our work on the film. We also appreciate the efforts of her agent William Reiss of John Hawkins and Associates, who worked so diligently on all our behalfs to bring this book to fruition.

The contribution of Mark O'Brien, whose life in the iron lung was the inspiration for the poetry included in this volume, helped to make this book unique. We hope that readers will be interested to see other pieces of Mark's poetry and will contact him through the Lemonade Factory at 1678 Shattuck Avenue, Suite 267, Berkeley, California 94709, or by calling (510) 548-2530.

Our own modest literary life would not have been achieved without the steady guidance and friendship of our agent Miriam Altschuler of the Miriam Altschuler Literary Agency. And this book could not have come to be without the support of our publisher at TV Books, Peter Kaufman, and his staff, particularly Joe Gannon and Keith Hollaman.

We owe equally heartfelt thanks to Tom Goodwin and Catherine Franklin of Porter Novelli, Inc., who helped us bring the film, the book, and the nationwide childhood immunization campaign so expertly and creatively to the American people.

Most of all, we owe thanks to our families: our respective spouses Ormond and Ellen, Minnesotans of great patience and tolerance, and our children, Aaron, Eleanor, Caleb, Casey, Frances, Daniel, and Mary Colleen. We can only look at them every day and be thankful that they will never be visited by the crippler poliomyelitis.

Nina Gilden Seavey and Paul Wagner
Takoma Park, Maryland and Charlottesville, Virginia
June, 1998

Introduction

We live in an age of enormous optimism about the conquest of disease. We also live in an age of dread. Better therapies extend the lives of HIV-positive patients, but as yet, there is no way to immunize against the virus that causes AIDS. Biologists develop ever more sophisticated ways of identifying those who may be susceptible to this or that obscure ailment, but too often cannot provide treatment for the dreaded condition whose arrival they can now predict. Advances in travel give us access to every quadrant of the globe, and diseases like the ebola virus or dengue fever migrate with appalling ease and speed. As we confront our fear of new diseases and struggle to find their causes and their cure, we look to past experience to help us prepare for the future.

Not very long ago, ours was a nation held hostage to terror. A fearful disease had come from nowhere, striking rich and poor, educated and ignorant, black and white. The victims lived in isolated rural communities, crowded cities, and pristine suburbs. The only thing they had in common was the tragic fact that most were children. The newly recognized danger was first called infantile paralysis, then poliomyelitis. As years passed and the number of victims rose, people came to call it polio—a short, urgent name for what seemed to be an inexorable menace. From the first large epidemic in 1916 to the introduction of the Salk vaccine in 1955 and the Sabin vaccine in 1961, the fear of polio was part of the pattern of American society, a dark thread woven through the fabric of national experience.

The story of polio is the story of how fear changed America. For over fifty years, no one could predict where or when the next epidemic would strike. No one could tell who would be hurt. No one knew what it was, or how it spread, or why it had arrived to attack the youngest, most innocent, most precious part of the population. No one had any idea how to prevent its terrible toll.

The first response was panic and distrust. Hospitals refused to treat the sick, neighbors fled from neighbors, schools and theaters closed for fear of contagion, ignorant doctors offered treatments that turned out to do more harm than good, and unscrupulous quacks profited from the desperation born from fear. Parents dreaded the small voice crying from bed, their child feverish, pain-wracked, and unable to move. They kept their children away from water fountains, swimming pools, sandboxes, city streets, summer camps, neighbors' houses, or wherever they thought contagion might lurk—but they could not keep out the fear that polio would seep through the cracks of their protection.

Polio could kill a child, and often did. But what made it such a vivid terror was the number of paralyzed victims who lived. In wheelchairs, on crutches, with arms or legs supported by metal braces or bodies encased in the dreaded iron lung, they were a constant reminder of the crippled, breathless aftermath of this most terrible plague. When people thought about polio, what they feared most was not death, but paralysis. To live in the age of polio was to live with a paralyzing fear.

And then, quite suddenly, it was over. In 1952, three years before the Salk vaccine was introduced, a new high of almost fifty-eight thousand cases of polio was reported in the United States alone. By 1960, despite delays in vaccination, incidence had dropped by 90 percent. After the widespread introduction of the Sabin vaccine, starting in 1961, polio cases in the United States fell to under ten per year. Today, polio is still found in developing nations, where access to health care is limited and interrupted, but there is hope that global immunization programs can eradicate the disease, perhaps as soon as within the next ten years.

The triumph over polio illustrates the best collaboration of science and public spirit. But there is another story here, as well. People must believe in the possibility of a cure before they can begin to seek one. They must believe in the value of the smallest child—not just as a potential contributor to the family economy, but as an infinitely precious promise to the future—before they can determine to make a childhood disease a medical priority. They must have confidence in mass movements before they will join one, and faith in authority before they will give their families over to a project such as the polio vaccine trials. The history of polio is not simply an account of medical triumph, though it is important to remember that part of the story. It is also an example of a society uniting to take action in the face of fear.

Some things seem eternal: distrust of the unknown, dread of contagion, reluctance to acknowledge the sick among us. The debates raging around the depiction of Franklin Roosevelt in the memorial recently installed in Washington show that there is still no consensus on the meaning or the portrayal of disability. Some things do change: for the first time in history we live in a society whose adults have little or no personal knowledge of the ravages of sudden epidemics and so they may underestimate their fearful power. Some things seem a tragic reenactment of the past: the struggle to control AIDS repeats many of the elements of the struggle to control polio, from the difficulty of funding research and treatment to the agonizing need to balance scientific testing against public demand for instant access to possible cures. We can only hope the conquest of AIDS is as happy and as fast as it was for polio.

The one certainty is that new terrors will always arise. Better medicines will come on the market and better research tools will be developed. We will continue to learn more about what steps we must take when confronting a new medical menace, whatever it may be. But scientific progress will never be enough. We must confront our fear before we can unite against its cause, and only from that process, with all its long, expensive, quarrelsome stages, can we hope to defeat disease.

The story of polio shows the worst and the best of American society. Epidemic diseases stun us with the numbers of people struck at once, but sickness strikes individuals, one by one. This dual perspective—public and private, national and individual, communal and very, very solitary—is captured on the following pages, as we move between the history of polio in America and the voices of individual polio survivors, who found themselves at the center of the crisis. In the end, it is a record of a triumphant national mobilization in a common cause, and of ordinary people caught up, most painfully, in extraordinary times. It is a story everyone should know.

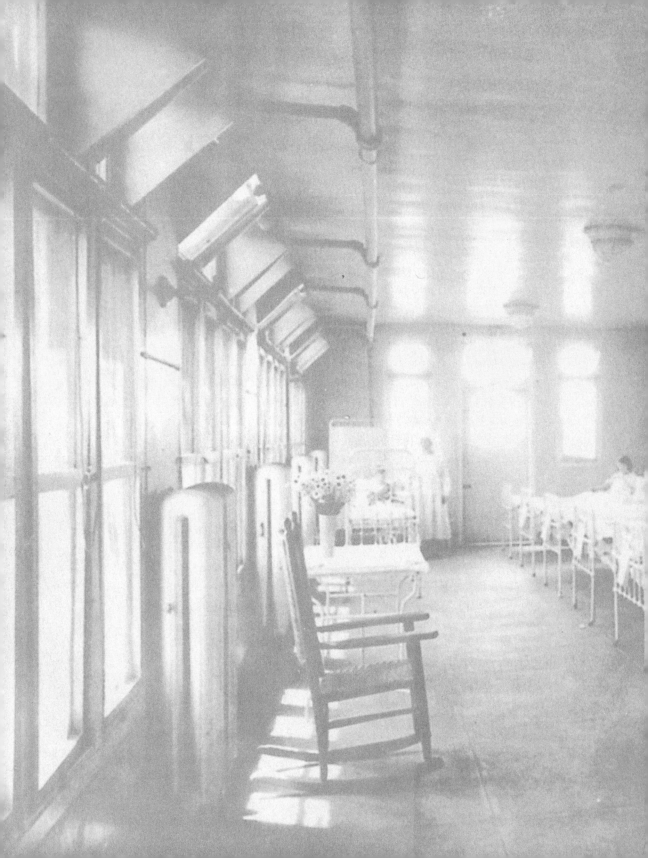

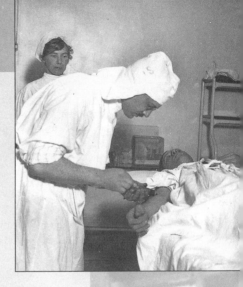

Chapter 1

New York, 1916

It was the robber of hope for a generation, several generations of children. There were diseases, and scientists will chart them, that were more devastating, affecting more children, more deadly than polio. But polio left kids crippled, and that was an image that this big strong postwar country simply couldn't abide. We had children lining up in wheelchairs, in iron lungs, whose very vitality and everyone's hope for their future was allayed right at the most critical time in their childhoods. And that's why polio seemed like such a horrible scourge, far more so than any number of other diseases or accidents that, any way you want to measure it, were more deadly and were fatal. And the image of a child in an iron lung is about as tearful and wrenching as we could imagine at that time, and any time certainly in this century. There were many other diseases that were bad for America, but polio broke its heart.

—Mark Sauer, polio survivor

America at the start of the century thought itself the most progressive place on earth. Not everybody enjoyed an equal share of peace and plenty, to be sure; many lives were bound by racial, national, and religious prejudice, and many people struggled to survive in desperate conditions of ignorance and want. But even among the poorest,

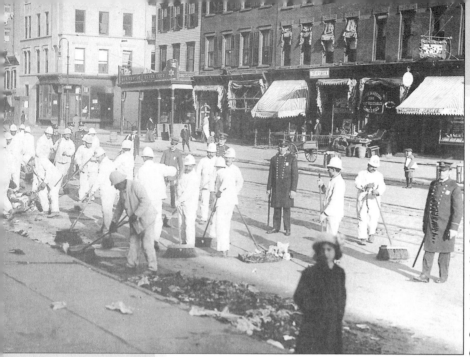

most Americans were confident that they lived in a time and place where opportunities were vast and individuals could shape their own destinies. And almost all agreed that science and technology would lead to man's conquest of disease and control over nature.

The evidence was all around them. Civil engineers were creating a network of aqueducts and water purification plants to provide clean, safe drinking water for much of the nation. Doctors trained in scientific diagnosis, rigorous hygiene, and modern medication were changing the practice of medicine from palliation to prevention and cure. The development of vaccines against cholera, tetanus, diphtheria, and rabies promised protection for what had been dreaded killers a generation before. Scientists like Louis Pasteur had discovered the bacterial sources of many infections, and other researchers were already positing the existence of something called viruses, disease agents so small they could not be seen under existing microscopes. Settlement houses, visiting nurse associations, municipal health departments, and other agencies of civic improvement dispatched nurses, doctors, and social workers to the poorest, least-educated sections of the community to bring principles of sanitation, nutrition, hygiene, and infant and child care to every family. Passage of the first Pure Food and Drug Act in 1902 promised added safety in food production and handling. Children from all walks of life were raised in the promise that the future would be better than the past.

Then, in the summer of 1916, tragedy struck. A mysterious epidemic began in New York City and stretched through the suburbs and countryside to the neighboring states of New Jersey, Pennsylvania, and Connecticut. Dozens, and then hundreds, and then thousands of children were taken ill. First the symptoms mimicked a cold, with a headache, often a chill, and then sometimes paralysis. The effect might be as mild as a stiff joint, or as severe as total paralysis of the arms, the legs, or even the whole body. For those whose muscles for breathing or swallowing were paralyzed, death came as suddenly as the mysterious disease itself. By mid-June, health officials realized they were dealing with a crisis; by mid-August almost nine thousand cases had been reported in the mid-Atlantic states. But what was it that was attacking so many children?

At first, nobody knew how to interpret the progress of the epidemic. Contagion was worse in Brooklyn and Staten Island than in Manhattan, but what did that mean? Victims in rural areas were more likely to die than those who lived in the more densely populated city, but what did that mean? Even the weakest elderly were less affected than the strongest child. What did that mean? No one could say.

Faced with mounting numbers of new cases, authorities responded by trying to repeat their recent successes against other epidemics. Scientific heroes like Pasteur and Joseph Lister had brought a new awareness of germs and of the value of cleanliness in preventing disease. Better sanitation in the home and in the community had steadily driven down the toll of killers like typhoid, dysentery, and tuberculosis, so New York City officials doused the streets with four million gallons of water a day and killed seventy-two thousand stray cats. Some officials advised quarantining families or entire districts. Oth-

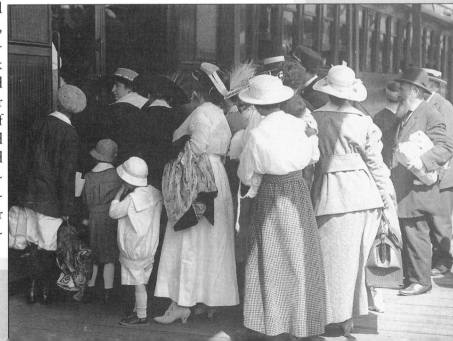

ers declared that only certain age groups, races, or nationalities were susceptible.

Decades would pass before researchers began to realize that polio epidemics were an ironic consequence of better sanitation, which kept infants from the early, mild infections that had generally conferred immunity in the past. In 1916, the idea that exposure to dirt might promote better health was too bizarre to imagine.

Confronted by evidence that contradicted most of what they knew about epidemic disease, public health authorities could not agree on the right approach...and the public knew it. Tempers flared, and contradictory recommendations fed a growing hysteria about the epidemic. Who was to blame? The early impulse was to blame the victim, and to try to prove that infection came from bad habits, poor hygiene, or poverty. New York City's slums teemed with immigrants from Italy and Eastern Europe. Their habits seemed strange and their neighborhoods were dirty. That middle-class New Yorkers who never went near the slums got polio made no difference. That Americans far from New York also got polio made no difference. Was it not possible that immigrants were harboring a new and terrible plague?

Looking back to the beginning of the century, it is easy to condemn the doctors and public health officials who claimed that the new paralysis was a product of poverty or moral degeneracy, or that it struck more heavily on one or another immigrant group precisely because of that group's "un-American" ways. What we have to remember is how helpless and threatened they felt. Faced with mystery, doctors and public officials had turned to science, and they had found no wisdom. It is sad but not surprising that, in the midst of terror that they, too, must have shared, the highest medical authorities slid into superstition and prejudice. The wonder is that it took so few decades to rise out of that abyss.

The first step was to identify the enemy. Studying autopsies in search of the nature of the epidemic, scientists named the new disease poliomyelitis, or inflammation of the anterior spinal cord. The public knew it as infantile paralysis—the disease that paralyzes infants. Smaller outbreaks had been noticed since the middle of the nine-

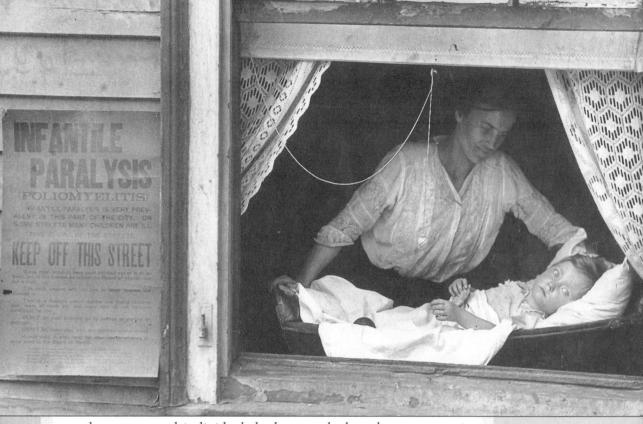

teenth century, and individuals had succumbed to the strange, crippling ailment for thousands of years, all over the world—but the number of people who showed any symptoms was so small that no one had ever even given a name to the affliction.

When the long summer of 1916 passed, the temperature dropped and so did the toll of poliomyelitis. By the end of the 1916 epidemic, twenty-seven thousand cases had been reported in twenty-six states, with six thousand deaths. Many milder cases undoubtedly went undiagnosed and unrecorded; epidemiologists now estimate that only one percent of polio cases led to the paralysis that is the disease's defining symptom. In New York City, where the epidemic was most fierce, there were 8,900 cases reported and 2,400 deaths between June and December of 1916. Eighty percent of the victims were children under five years old.

The terrors of the 1916 polio epidemic were soon eclipsed by the brutal horrors of World War I and by the staggering death toll (over 600,000 people in the United States alone) of the influenza pandemic of the fall of 1918. Yet there was a difference that made 1916

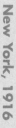
New York, 1916

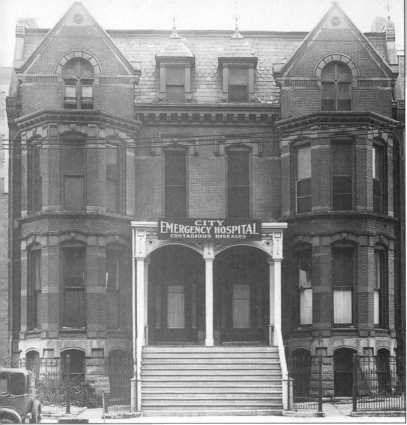

memorable. Unlike the victims of war or influenza, most of the children who had been struck by polio survived. They were left with withered arms, useless legs, or twisted backs, but they were still very much alive, visible reminders of the mysterious crippler that had assaulted the metropolis and the nation. They lurched about on heavy wooden crutches, were wheeled in homemade wagons, limped on shoes with elevated soles, or, quite often, were left to languish at home, unwelcome by the society of the able-bodied.

There were few provisions for their care. Orthopedic surgeons struggled to devise ways to deal with paralysis and physical distortion, but the world was unprepared for a sudden generation of crippled children. Those who needed special care, and could afford it, lived in places with terrible names like "The Home for Incurables" or "The Hospital for the Ruptured and Crippled." The wealthy could buy wheelchairs and hire private nurses to care for polio survivors, but there was little they could do to improve their condition.

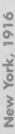

New York, 1916

Voices
Marilyn Rogers

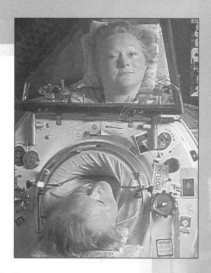

Marilyn Rogers was nine years old when she came down with polio that affected the use of her limbs and her respiratory muscles. She has lived either in an iron lung or on a respirator since 1949.

What are your first memories of having polio?

I was nine years old and it was 1949. I had this tremendous headache and my back hurt. That was when my cousin came over to check me out and she tried to touch my hand to my knees and I couldn't do it. And she decided to call the doctor. We met the doctor at the hospital and [he] told me they would do a test for polio, that I would have to curl up on the table with my back up to get a spinal tap. And he said it would hurt. He said he was going to put some Novocain in, which he did. And I had to push against it with my back because it wouldn't go in. And I do not recall it hurting. He did a good job. He told my mother that I had a really high cell count and that I should be in the hospital. So I was placed in a room with three or four other children. We had this horrendous outfit to put on, pajama bottoms and a top that was open on the back. And I noticed all of the other children had bandages on their backs. That's a real vivid memory. And I thought, 'Gee I must have one too.'

The next morning I was having difficulty moving and sitting up. I remember picking up my glass of chocolate milk and it fell through my hands. And they came in and I couldn't have any more chocolate milk. I later learned that it was because they thought I might choke on it. My headache was getting worse. I was getting a lot of pain in my limbs. And the doctors started coming in having me count backwards from ten to one, and at some point I was not able to do it, so they told me they could put me in a machine to make me feel better, easier to breathe. They took me into a small room. I saw this giant machine. To me it was giant. And they had to slide it open. There was a tray inside. They put me on I, slid my head through. I thought it was silly at the time because it took three people to carry me. I think they were trying to keep from bending my back. I remember when they turned it on. I felt comfortable. I could breathe. They told me it was unusual because most people fought it, I guess. I remember there was a chest of drawers across the room. It had gladiolas on it.

The hospital had eighty patients in iron lungs. I do remember the power failure a few times. The first time I passed out and they just grabbed everybody, then the power would go back on. It got so that I panicked when it went off because I couldn't breathe.

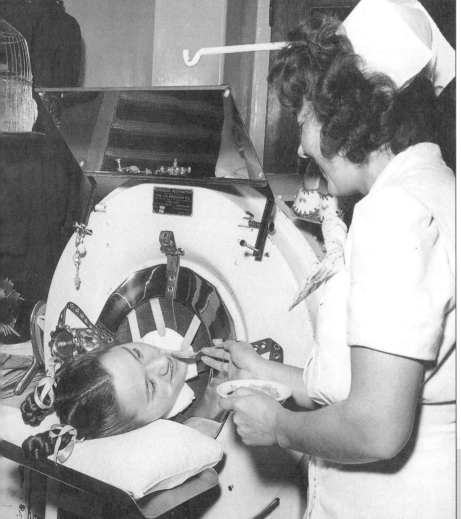

What was going through your head at age nine being on this machine?

Staying alive. The staff were very, very nice to us. Some of the nurses that they called 'plague nurses' at the National Foundation, they were the best. One of them brought peas in with straws so that we could see if we could hit the ceiling to increase our vital capacity. I usually give nicknames to everybody. She wore purple fingernail polish. So I called her 'Purple.'

What else do you remember about being at Minneapolis General?

I was a dancer and I'd been to school since I was three. Everybody said I had talent but I wasn't sure. I was very athletic. I guess it said on my chart that I danced and one of the physicians wanted to . . . he just twirled me around the floor. He wasn't a very good dancer. But that was the last time I danced.

What happened after those initial months?

At that time Sister Kenny would not take anybody that had been in an iron lung. The recovery rate was not quite as good. So the doctors, along with the National Foundation, said they would stop funding patients if she didn't take us. There were no spots left in any other hospitals by the time they got to the irons. So I remember one day they sent me to the hospital. They met us at the door and said [my mother and father] couldn't come in, which was really frightening because I was wondering what the hell was going to happen here. I was really frightened without my parents. My parents were allowed to see me two hours on Sunday. When before that I was used to anytime. My father used to come in the middle of the night at the old hospital, the first hospital.

What happened when you first arrived at Sister Kenny?

I remember being taken to a room and some other doctor checked me over. I wasn't used to being out of the respirator for long periods of time. So I was getting tired. I wanted to go back in the respirator. And they didn't put me on at first. I think it was several hours. I was really exhausted. I just went to sleep after I got there.

I had a cloth around my neck, to keep my neck from getting rubbed away by the collar. And one day it was starting to hurt, and it slid [so that] I couldn't breathe. It took at least two people to fix it. So people had to work fast. I was crying and called the nurse. You had to learn to really melt to get her attention. She came in and she seemed really frustrated, overworked, and just too busy. So I told her what was wrong and she just told me to stop crying. She said she would turn my respirator off if I didn't stop crying. When she did I passed out immediately. My friend Allison, who was next to me, told me what went on. It saddened some assistants and they turned it back on. I didn't

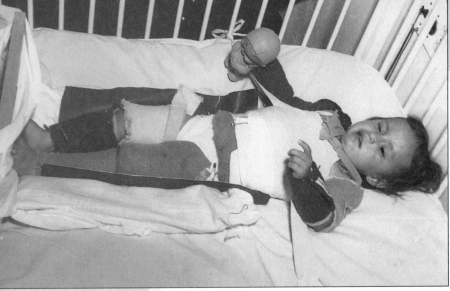

say anything because I was too afraid. By morning my neck was worn away down to the bone and my mother came so I told her. I trusted her. I never saw the nurse again. I assumed they fired her. But it took months and months and months for it to heal because I had to be in the respirator.

That was really a pivotal point for me because I was now afraid of what was going to happen to me. I was taken from a familiar hospital to a non-familiar hospital. Some of the staff at Sister Kenny were a little sadistic. I think they kind of gravitated to a plague like that when the public isn't in and out like that all the time. So when I had people coming to work I never knew what they were going to be like that day. It was really hard so I had to adjust to each person, each personality. That was difficult. So I've noticed now I can adhere only to people that don't seem controlling over me. That is a real issue for me. I need to control my environment. So I don't have to adjust to a different person every day.

I was at Sister Kenny's for two years. I was able to be out of the respirator for a little while at that time. Unless I was sick I would usually get out of the bed to feed myself. I figured out a way to set up my plate so that I could use one hand a little bit to feed myself. Then we usually had g-strings on all the time. It seems rather weird but in bed we wore gowns. Once in a while we would get clothes on—I think when visitors would come. We had therapy, which consisted of putting plaster under each part of my body, wrapping it in hot pads: shoulders, upper arm, lower arm, hands, chest, hips, thighs, calves, feet. It was really hot. They did that maybe two to three times a day. One day I was asking a packer that put the hot packs on to please stop because it was just so hot. I had a brilliantly red chest.

Did you make friends?

Some of my friends were adults and some were children. I think everyone was under a lot of stress, so it wasn't really a normal situation. I think we either got to know each other very well or not at all. Some kids clammed up. I remember I had just gotten a new pair of ice skates just before I got polio. One of the kids wanted my skates because I was giving them away. And I don't know why she kept them because she wasn't going to be able to use them. I always thought that was strange.

How did you keep your spirits up?

While I was a kid I didn't want to live. I was really tired of not seeing my parents. So for awhile I just didn't want to be around. I stopped eating and drinking. I couldn't do it any faster. And the doctor came in one day and said, 'You've got to start eating and drinking, one way or the other. You know what's going to happen?' I said, 'Yes.' He said, 'I'd really like you to start drinking.' I said, 'Well, only if my parents can come and see me more often.' He said, 'That could probably be arranged.' And I said, 'Could they bring a meal in?' Home cooked food was really missing. The food was pretty bad. So he relented. After that I also stated that, 'I'd like it if other people's parents could come too, more often.' So it happened. It was my first political move and I liked the power.

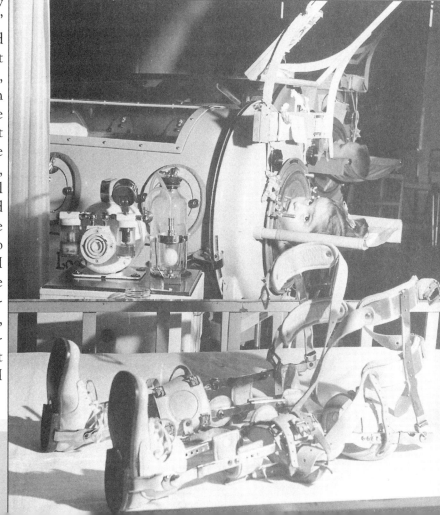

What was the prevailing attitude at Sister Kenny?

The doctor kind of projected the attitude that those of us in iron lungs were not going to be worth much if we had to go home with an iron lung. The emphasis was on being on twenty-four hours a day for the rest of your life. The National Foundation finally changed their mind on this—to let us go home with iron lungs. When I was in both hospitals the National Foundation paid for everything. My parents were not able to pay. So I felt obligated later when everyone wanted stories. They were using me to elicit sympathy so people would part with their money. To me that attitude prevails. Pity versus cold respect.

Tell me about your birthday at Sister Kenny.

That was really interesting. My parents had arranged to bring cake and ice cream for everybody on the ward. I remember getting these presents that I thought, 'Why am I getting these? I can't play with them.' It was just a real hard experience because I was more realistic than they were. My friends and parents and stuff gave me gifts, like dolls to play with, puzzles. I told my parents to give them to the other kids.

Tell me about going home, which was two and a half years after you left.

I had to spend five weeks out of the respirator first. They had done that twice to try to see if I could survive. I was loony—lack of sleep, I guess, 'cause I would really drift instead of sleeping. My mother was there, the doctor came in and said that I could go home because my parents were assisting. The National Foundation allowed me to go home and they actually paid for a nurse. We called it a nurse, but I had who I wanted to stay while my parents worked. They used to say to my mom, 'You know, she is not going to live past six months if you take her home.' And I knew differently. She was quite upset that I left.

I remember being taken home. It was just great. I wanted to go by car but they wanted me to go by ambulance. I got in the house. It had changed because the bed was in the dining room. That was the only available room. They didn't want me upstairs in a bedroom. That was silly. And there was a bay window right beside my bed. It was not very private but in that house you learned to ignore privacy because you didn't have any. My brother—I had to get reacquainted with him. He had to get reacquainted with me. There were family to come over, relatives who lived around the city. I had a giant meal. I loved the food. It was great. My old friends came over to visit me one evening, kids my age. They seemed the same. I'd changed. I was kind of an adult after that. I didn't think we had anything in common anymore. It was strange. For them, too. They had no way of relating to me. I couldn't play sports anymore. I was really a ham before. I would put on these shows and force them to watch them. That had totally changed. So after that most of my friends were adults. I dealt with life and death issues in watching people survive.

How did you go about your education?

I didn't have any education at the first hospital. When I was at Kenny they had a teacher. Ha ha, teacher. She was interested in doing crafts, which I couldn't do. She did some teaching but very little. My brain was going stale. I finished the third grade before I got polio. Then I started the fourth grade. So I skipped the fourth, fifth, sixth, and seventh grades because there was no teaching from public schools

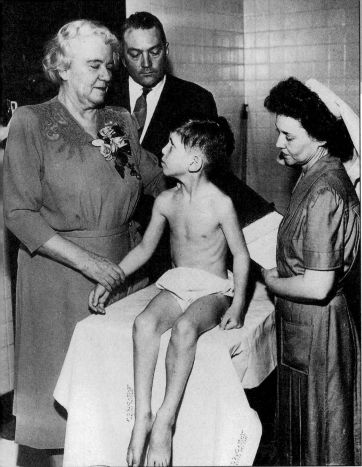

unless I could go there. They said I couldn't. In the very early 1960s they started programs for unwed mothers. They had home teaching, so that program transferred over to people who were disabled. So I got a teacher for four hours a day once a week. I had to catch up, plus go on. I think I skipped a lot of my education. The curriculum was confined by what they taught at my local school. I wanted to take Latin and they wouldn't give it to me. That was really frustrating. I wanted to take a lot of courses that were restricted.

Can you tell me about the special chair your father made for you?

They sent me home from the hospital with a regular wheelchair, and I could sit for a little while but I'd pass out because my butt hurt so much and I got tired. So he thought of putting a lawn chair with wheels, taking a lawn chair and putting wheels on it, which was perfect. Then I could recline. I could move around and be comfortable and do the things I wanted to do.

What happened the first time you went out in public?

Well, the first time I used the wheelchair they sent me home with, the nurse was pushing me down the street and this old man saw me and started walking backwards, saying, 'Oh, you poor thing, you poor thing, what happened to you?' And I got really angry, really upset. I came home and told my parents I was never going out again. My mother said, 'How close was he to you?' And I said he was pretty close and she said, 'You could spit in his eye.' I said, 'Yeah, I could.' And my father and mother both said, 'Well, you are going to have to face that or lead the rest of your life in the house.' So I chose to be out doing things.

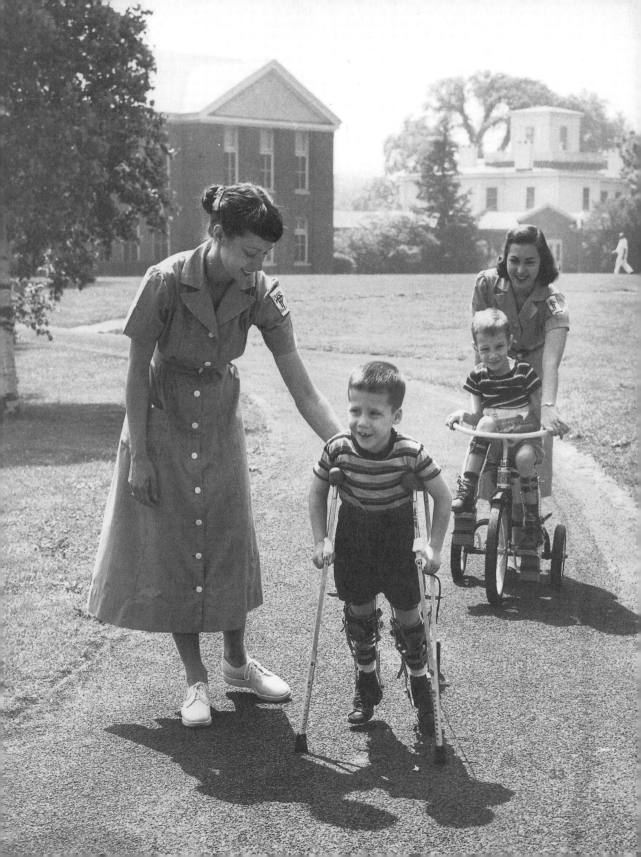

And today you go out. Tell me about your day now.

Oh, my day now, that's boring, let's talk about back then, all the trips I've been on. Boring, boring, boring. I wake up in the morning about maybe 6:30 and I stay in the respirator now for most of the morning because I've got asthma. If I don't have too much congestion, I get out about 12:00 to 1:00. Then I can do things, go downtown, go to different events, if I'm able to. I usually stay out 'til really late, going to jazz clubs.

Tell me about your most memorable trip.

My most memorable trip is the first time I went to Seattle to see the rest of my family, to get reacquainted. It was really nice and I stayed at my brother's house. The first trip was really memorable to me. I went to San Diego to visit another brother, he was in the Navy. My parents and I and a friend went. That was when I was still taking the lawn chair, because they still didn't have reclining wheelchairs. We went every day, I was astonished at how accessible things were. I could get to places there that I couldn't even get to in my own home town, curb cuts everywhere, ramps, I could get into museums, I could go to cultural events, music, plus just get around the city to sightsee. We drove down to Mexico. That was fun.

Eleanor Tafil, R.N.

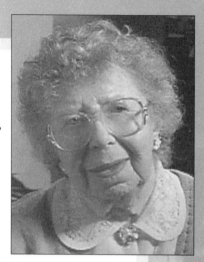

Eleanor Tafil was a nurse who treated polio patients from the 1930s through the 1950s in Seattle, Washington. She remembers the day she assisted in the birth of a child from a woman confined to an iron lung.

Could you tell me your recollections of the 1932 epidemic?

I was in training at Children's Hospital, what was then called the Orthopedic hospital. It was 1933, and they had had the polio epidemic the year before. There were wards of little children on metal frames if their back was curbed. Little children are wonderful patients. They don't realize that they have this terrible thing, that they're never going to walk again, so our job, besides taking care of them, was entertaining them, keeping them happy. And at that time they felt that when parents visited all the time it upset the children, so parents only came Sunday afternoon. Then Sunday evening all the children had temperatures because they'd been worked up by that. So it was all up to the nurses, and of course they were all student nurses and some volunteers.

In 1932 you couldn't do very much for the children.

When you think back then, they didn't even have vitamins. We would go around and give cod liver oil to each child. There wasn't anything else to do other than massage them and exercise their legs, offer skin care, and entertain them. I suppose these are the children that became cripples. I went back to the hospital, back to Children's in the 1950s, and that was the very end of polio. Then they were doing the Kenny treatment, and anyone who worked with them can remember that smell of wet wool. We would have the arm or the leg and we would have these pieces of old wool blanket that were in these wet, hot, steamy machines. We would take them out and wrap them around the patient. And between that, you would massage. The terrible wasting of the muscles hadn't started yet. So there was always hope. You always would try to get them to move. You know, 'Can you move your toes?' 'Can you move your arm or hand?'

How did the children respond to the wet wool treatment?

They would fuss about it. But the younger they were, the more they would take for granted. The older the children were, the more angry they were. Because by that time they realized, 'I can't move my arm' or 'I can't move my leg.' Where the little ones didn't seem to notice that. 'Course, I always said I never took care of an adult that I could hold in my lap and rock and they would feel better. You could do that with a child.

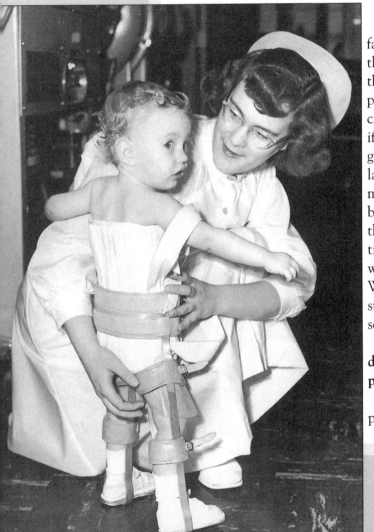

What role did parents play?

Mothers were better than fathers—they would never show their discouragement in front of their child. Because the child would pick up if mamma was sitting there crying and they'd be frightened. But if mamma would laugh and play games with them, the child would laugh and play games. I've seen mothers who would hate to go home because they would be so afraid their child would be crying all the time. But they had to because there were other children [at home]. When mother left then we would step in and take over. And they seemed to know the routine.

What did you do with the children while they were in the hospital?

We read to them. And we would push their beds all together for

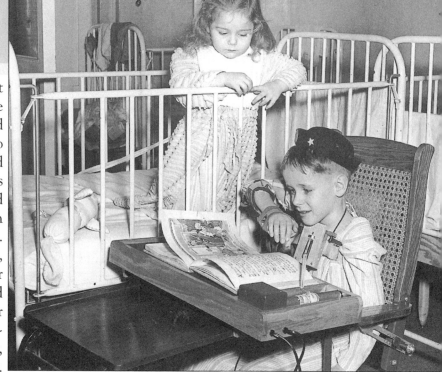

entertainment, so that they could see. In the winter when it snowed we'd pull all the beds to the window. In fact, we'd go out on the big porches and make snowballs and bring it in so the children could hold the snowballs. If they were old enough, we had a school teacher who came around, and we'd help them do their homework. And if anyone had a birthday, why, there was a big party. We'd have a cake and candles. Every ward had a big room that we could pull the beds to, like a living room, and if they happened to be there for Christmas, why, Santa Claus came around. We hung up the stockings on everyone's bed at night, and Santa Claus came around and gave them presents. I worked many Christmases, so with my own children we'd have our Christmas on Christmas Eve so that I could be at the hospital on Christmas. I'd go around with Santa Claus, and you know, 'Ho, ho, ho.' And I can remember a child might say, 'I was afraid you wouldn't see me here.' And Santa would say, 'Why, I couldn't miss you.' So a lot was done for the children. I think in many cases it was harder on the parents. I mean, anyone who is a parent can imagine what it would be to think that your child wasn't going to be home for a birthday or for Christmas.

Did some children get better enough to walk again?

Yes. We had a physical therapy department who would take them down and they would be fitted for braces. And the first time we saw a spinal jack fusion, we couldn't believe our eyes. It looked like the doctor had gone to the hardware store and said, 'Well, I'll take some of that and some of that' and put it in. Nowadays we're used to having metal pieces in us. But children are always so hopeful. I can remember putting a child in braces from the hips down to their toes and having them stand up and say, 'Oh it's so nice to be standing up,' even though they were standing up with braces and crutches. It was a thrill to them, to be in that position.

Could you talk about how parents reacted to a child in the iron lung?

Well, they were terrified. But we warned them, and they were very good with the children. If a little child was in an iron lung it was, 'Oh, look at the funny house you're in.' No one would say, 'This is a terrible thing that you're in.' You couldn't even think of that.

What happened to the pregnant woman who got polio?

That was the one time that it really struck me how devastating polio could be. I was working on the OB floor in Seattle General, and we heard that a mother in labor was coming in. And we were sort of shocked when she was brought up in a wheelchair. Not our wheelchair, in her own little wheelchair. And she was a mother who had polio. She couldn't use her legs. So we timed her pains and everything else that you do. It was when we got her in the delivery room, and we had to put her legs up in stirrups, that we realized how devastating it can be. It was almost as if she had no bones in her legs. The muscles were so gone from the hip down. And we ended up having to tie her legs in because we couldn't control them otherwise. It was a fairly difficult delivery and I thought that poor little mother, having to take care of her children from a wheelchair.

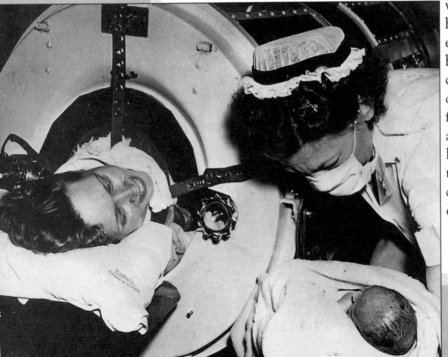

Josephine Howard

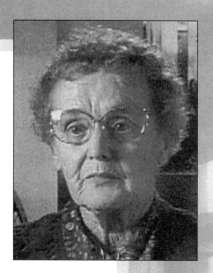

Josephine Howard is the matriarch of the
Howard family of Lodi, California. Her
daughters Eleanor, Charlotte, Linda, and
Patti were all stricken by the disease and her
son, Richard, died of polio. Her husband,
Rufus, also contracted the disease the day
after Richard's funeral and spent the rest of
his life managing the family farm from his
wheelchair.

Can you tell me about your family, and which members got polio?

I had six children. Richard got it first and then Patty, Linda, then
Charlotte and Eleanor. And then my husband Rufus got it, fourteen
days after the others.

**Mrs. Howard, I'd like to go back and talk a little bit about
Richard. I know that's the hardest part.**

Well, he looked so much better from when I brought him in. He had
color and it was a relief to me to think he might be improving. But
from there he had to go into the lung. I brought him in with a homemade quilt and they put him in the oxygen and then they let me see
him. I came to the door and I'm holding the quilt. And when I saw
him I started to cry, and the attendant said to me, 'Oh, that's a beautiful quilt,' his way of sort of soothing me a little bit. They'd let us go
see him in the lung and we'd sit outside and listen to the pumping.
Then they'd say, 'You need to go home, there's no change.' And they'd
call us and we'd come back again and go see him and wait. But actually we were not with him when he passed away.

Tell me about his funeral.

Well, the funeral. My husband and I had to go buy him a little outfit. So we went to the children's store and picked out a pretty little

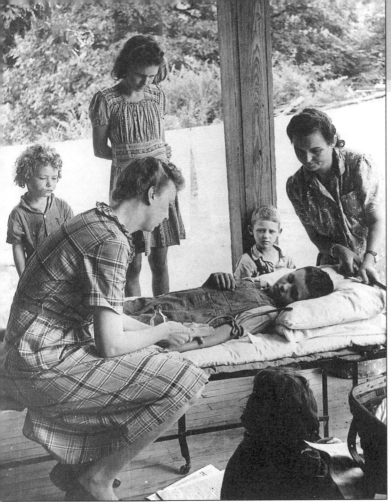

blue suit, and the lady said the legs were long and said, 'Oh that's okay, he'll grow into them.' And my husband and I, neither one of us said anything. What do you say? It would make the poor lady feel bad. The funeral was small because we didn't want people to come. But my sister came and tried to give Rufus a hug and he said, 'Don't touch me.' We didn't know how it was passed on. And the next day he became ill. He had a carbuncle on the back of his neck, so the doctor put him in the hospital. The next morning they made us come immediately because they found out it was involved in polio. They didn't give him any crutches or wheelchair and he was already losing the use of his leg. So we went down in the elevator and we had a neighbor there who was going to help me. And Rufus said, 'No way, go away, don't touch me.' So I put him in the back seat of the car and took him down to French Camp, where the girls were, and of course we found out he did have it too.

Tell me a little about the girls coming home.

Linda came home first. She was only in there for one month, and she had the same type as Richard. Her eye wouldn't close good and her mouth was a little crooked. But all I could do was to get my family back piece by piece, which was wonderful. My mom was there to help me because I had to give them treatments when they came home, every night a hot bath, manipulate the legs, and Linda's little face, we would work with it too. The others didn't come home for two more months,

Charlotte and Patty. Eleanor was ill at home but never had the real paralysis.

How did your family cope?

Christmas wasn't easy because the little one wasn't there. But we did fine, because they were young enough to appreciate Christmas in a child's way. So we had a tree, dinner, and the whole thing. And my husband came home just for Christmas because he didn't come home until April. At first they allowed Rufus to come home maybe once a week. So then he would come home and there was no use of his left leg and his shoulder muscles were real bad. So he'd have the hired man put him on the tractor. Then he would go back to the hospital. So he would want to work more and wouldn't get to the hospital on time, so finally he just scratched it and stayed home and farmed. And worked in the shop. At first he had his crutches and later he had a wheelchair, and he could weld, fix machines, and take a tractor apart and put it all together, and when he had crutches he would walk the farm on crutches. He did anything that needed doing. He was an amazing person.

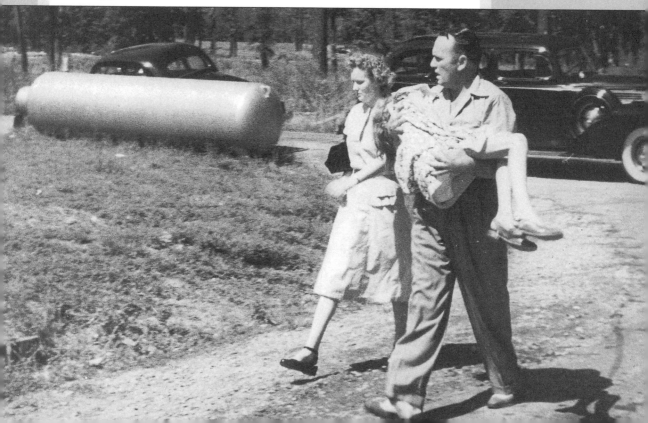

How did people react to your family?

The lady in the hospital who came around to see everyone said it was because I didn't clean the vegetables. That was why my family had polio, which, of course, was not true at all. One day, I had taken the crib out on the front porch and I was washing it. I was supposed to wash the bedroom top to bottom with Clorox. And the gas man came to fill the barrels and he said, 'Oh, hi, Mrs. Howard, how are you this morning?' And he asked what I was doing. I explained the whole situation with polio, and he threw his arms up and said, 'Oh my goodness,' and he left. And I think part of it was because he had two children of his own, and that's understandable, but it did make you feel rather strange and lonely.

What about your neighbors, did they come help you?

The elderly ones. This little Italian lady Mrs. Tucci came and she helped me wash clothes and fold clothes and just be with me, but she wouldn't let her daughter-in-law come because she was younger. And it was like that in the whole neighborhood. We were pretty isolated because people didn't want to come around, you know. How did they know where it came from?

How did you react when the vaccine came out?

I wished the vaccine had come out earlier. It was just a few years. We had it in 1946 and the vaccine was early 1950s. We went and had the shot anyway.

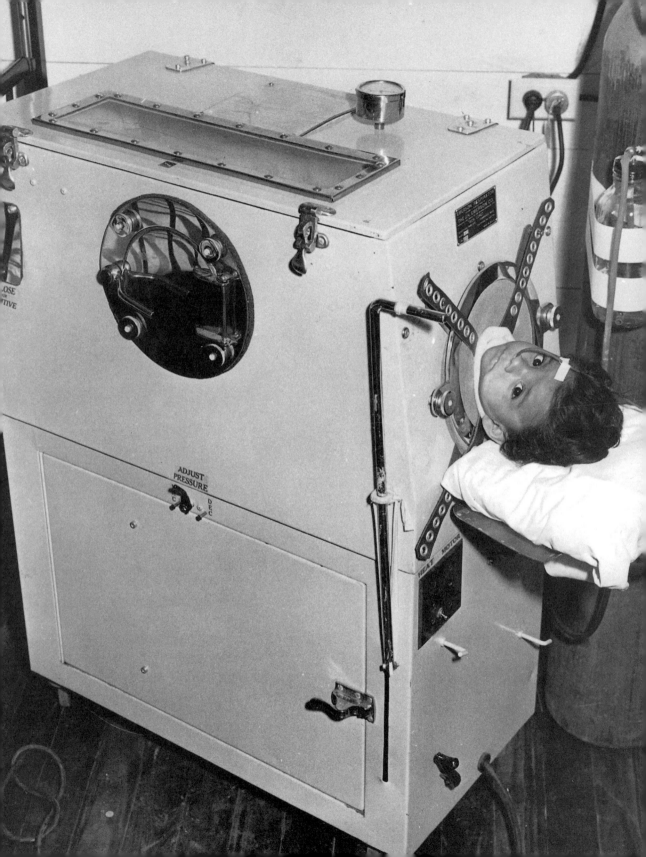

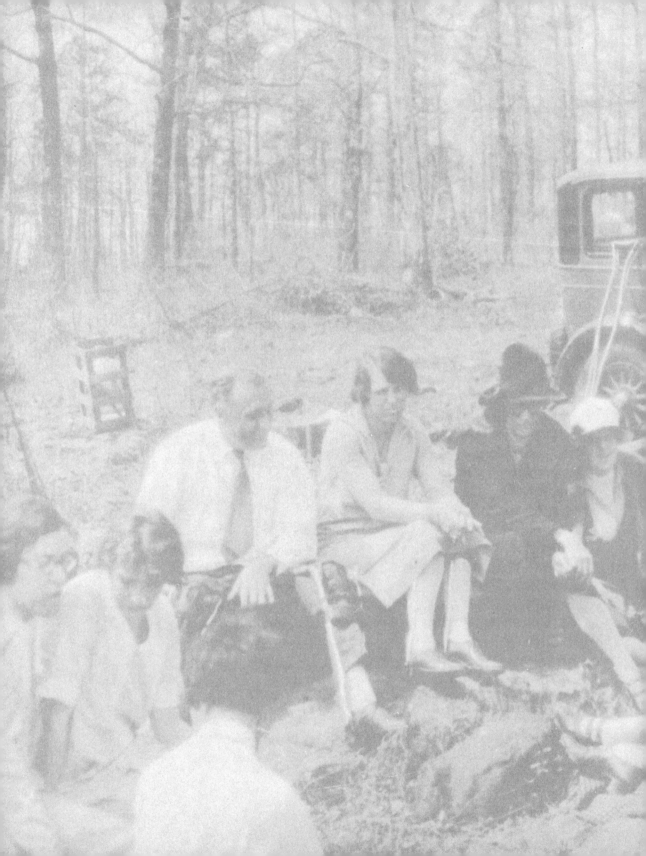

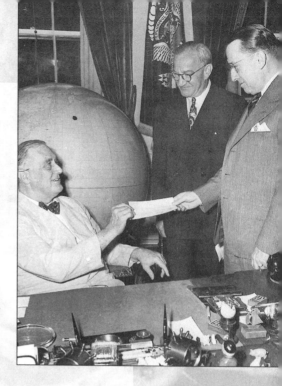

Chapter 2

FDR and the Transformation of Polio

> Polio changed FDR. He had had a life of unparalleled
> success until then. He was an only son and his mother
> adored him, showered him with attention. He had always
> been given anything he wanted. And then he got polio.
> Polio was the only thing that he had ever confronted that
> he couldn't beat. He had decided, 'I'm going to lick this,
> I'm going to walk again.' And seven years of his life were
> devoted entirely to rehabilitation. And he didn't win.
> He was no more rehabilitated at the end of seven years
> than he was at the beginning.
>
> —Hugh Gallagher, polio survivor and
> biographer of Franklin Roosevelt

It would take a very famous victim to concentrate the energy of a nation on finding a way to end the polio epidemics. In August 1921, on a wooded island off the coast of Maine, a man fell ill and the fate of polio was forever changed.

Despite its common name, infantile paralysis, not every victim of poliomyelitis was an infant, or even a child. Franklin Delano Roosevelt was thirty-nine years old, the father of five children, and a rising star in Democratic national politics when he succumbed to the virus. He had served as Under-Secretary of the Navy during World War I and had been nominated for Vice President in 1920. The Democrats had lost that election, but Roosevelt had emerged with a national reputation. Wealthy, handsome, ambitious, and well-connected to the inner circles of both social and political power, he seemed destined for a smooth and effortless rise into elected office. But on August 11, 1921, while vacationing with his family at their summer home on Campobello Island, New Brunswick, he felt an unfamiliar fatigue that drove him to his bed. Over the few days it took the disease to progress from chills to lethargy to paralysis, Roosevelt's life was transformed, and with it the history of polio in America.

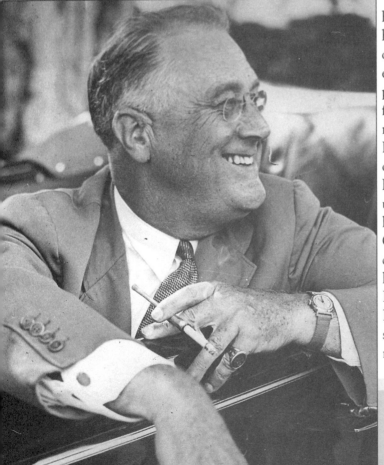

Roosevelt was already exhausted when he fell ill. He had hoped to spend the entire summer on Campobello Island, a remote enclave of rustic country houses popular with wealthy society families, but he had been forced to rush to sweltering Washington, D.C., to defend himself against an old Navy scandal that the new Republican administration was using to discredit him. From there he traveled by train to New York City, where he found himself delayed by business. On July 25, he escaped the city to attend a Boy Scout rally at New York's Bear Mountain Park, on the Hudson River, and ten days later he made a harrowing, storm-delayed return by private yacht to Campobello. Somewhere along the way, Roosevelt had already picked up the polio virus.

Tired from his travels but glad to be back at the family retreat, Roosevelt took his children sailing on August 10. They swam in the icy Atlantic water, then landed to help fight a forest fire on shore. Still in a wet bathing suit, Roosevelt read through his mail. He felt chilled and went to bed. The next morning, he awoke with an odd weakness in his right knee. That evening the left knee gave way. By the following morning he could not use his legs. Franklin Roosevelt never walked again unassisted.

Roosevelt was able to call the best doctor from Boston to his bedside, but while Robert Lovett was able to confirm the diagnosis, he knew as little as anyone else about how to treat poliomyelitis. Sara Roosevelt, who dominated the entire family and doted on her only son, felt he should return to her home in Hyde Park, New York, to spend the rest of his life as a genteel invalid. Roosevelt's wife Eleanor disagreed. So did his gruff, canny political advisor, Louis Howe. Between them, they managed to convince the world that Franklin Roosevelt's paralysis was only a temporary setback to his political progress, a career that he might resume at any time.

At first, however, and for many months thereafter, Roosevelt's main interest was in his physical recovery. For much of the next seven years, Roosevelt devoted most of his time and energy, and a good deal of his personal fortune, on efforts to regain the use of his legs. He tried heat, massage, exercise, electric currents, and anything else that sounded even faintly promising. In 1924, at the suggestion of George Foster Peabody, a friend and well-known philanthropist, Roosevelt visited Warm Springs, Georgia, a thermal spa for the well-to-do, whose waters were rumored to "cure" paralysis.

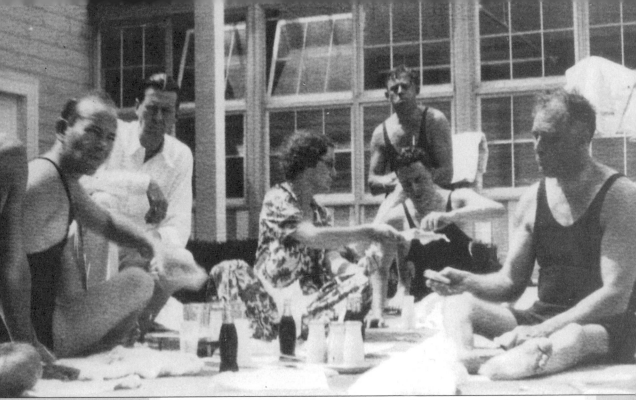

The resort at Warm Springs had been losing business for years and was badly in need of repair, and Peabody's recommendation may well have been influenced by the fact that he was the owner. Eleanor Roosevelt judged Warm Springs "derelict," and was disturbed by segregated and unprogressive social conditions in the surrounding area. Louis Howe thought Franklin should be spending time closer to the centers of political action and less on his unprofitable investments and unsuccessful cures. But Roosevelt was convinced that swimming in the naturally heated pools helped his condition. Aided by the buoyant water, he began to invent a series of water exercises. They did nothing to end his paralysis, but the exercise did build up other muscles and made him feel better. Captivated by Warm Springs, Roosevelt spent over half his personal fortune to buy the property in 1926.

Thanks to Louis Howe, Roosevelt's name continued to appear in the news, and many reports noted his "water cure" at Warm Springs. Soon other polio patients were arriving to try "Doctor" Roosevelt's warm water spa. Frightened by these living reminders of a disease whose causes and cures were still entirely unknown, guests who were not recovering from polio soon abandoned the resort. Those who were left formed their own society. They called themselves "polios," and they stayed on at Warm Springs long after they could pay their bills. Here, no one felt ashamed or self-conscious about paralysis. The very existence of Warm Springs gave them hope.

As history's most prominent and charismatic "polio," Roosevelt did more than any other person to change the popular image of the disease from something shameful and dirty to what it was: a sometimes debilitating infection that could, and did, strike anyone. Still, Roosevelt also made sure the public never saw the true extent of his paralysis. In 1928, when he decided to run for governor of New York State, Roosevelt applied for an insurance policy, complete with a thorough physical examination, to counter rumors that the candidate was too frail to govern. As the doctors' reports were spread throughout the newspapers, the public learned that Roosevelt had lost most of the use of his legs, but was otherwise in vigorous health. It was more than a political assurance. It was an education for the public in not defining people by their disability. Polio survivors might have a crippled an arm or leg, but they were not weak or powerless.

Roosevelt never did recover from his initial paralysis, yet to the public he seemed to walk. During public appearances he locked his leg braces so his knees would not buckle. He leaned on a cane, or on someone's arm, and he thrust himself forward— held up by steel, propelled by will. His paralysis was not a secret; it had been announced on page one of *The New York Times*, but it was never allowed to be a visible trait. For the rest of his life, Roosevelt allowed no photographs of himself being carried or wheeled about. It was an era when journalists wanted to help create the image of a strong leader, not expose

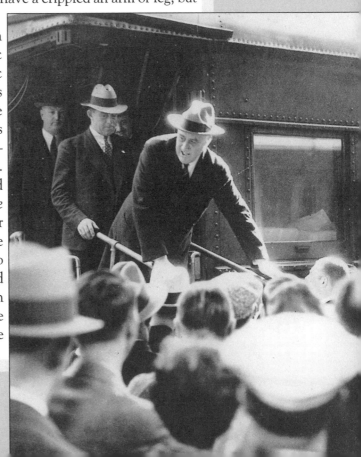

the weaknesses of those in power, and the press cooperated. When the public saw Roosevelt sitting behind a desk, or in a car, or leaning forward against a railing to address a crowd, they saw a figure of command, mobility, and passion. Only two private photos are known to exist of Roosevelt in his wheelchair.

Roosevelt's four terms in the White House created a lasting change in American attitudes toward all the survivors of this still mysterious disease. The President of the United States had had polio, but he was busy now leading the world's most powerful nation out of the Depression and toward victory in World War II. In serving as a model for the polio survivor and as a person of vigor who merely happened to be unable to walk, Roosevelt created many new opportunities for all people with disabilities; it was only much later that people would begin to question the other aspect of Roosevelt's model, the assumption that patients were supposed to overcome their injuries by hiding them.

For the portion of the public that shared Roosevelt's paralysis, the vibrant image he projected was a difficult, and probably impossible, goal. In truth, Roosevelt himself couldn't live up to his public role as the perfect polio survivor. He concealed his pain and created a vast conspiracy around him to hide the extent of his paralysis. The polio survivors, seeing the newsreels, didn't know that, however. They only knew that they should try as hard as possible and they, too, might be President.

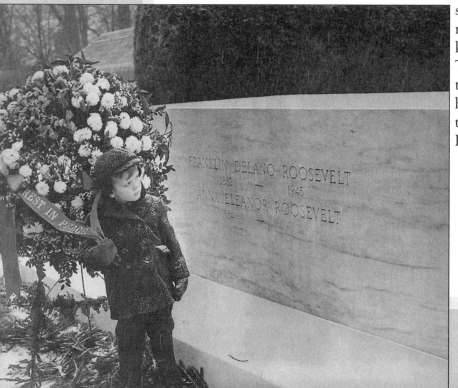

Voices
Hugh Gallagher

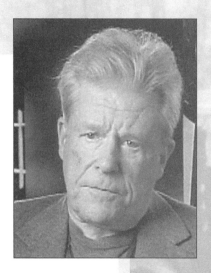

Hugh Gallagher had just been accepted
to join an expedition to go to the North
Pole overland via dogsled when he contracted polio at age nineteen. He was confined to an iron lung for eight weeks and
never did regain the use of his legs. He
underwent rehabilitation at Warm Springs,
Georgia, and ultimately wrote a biography
of FDR, entitled *FDR's Splendid Deception*,
about Franklin Roosevelt's relationship with
his disease and its aftermath.

**Go back to when you were nineteen and you knew there was
something wrong.**

It was 1952, and I was a sophomore at Haverford College just outside of Philadelphia. I had broken loose from my family, and had broken loose from a school that I had hated, MIT. On my own I had
sought admission to Haverford, and this was my first semester, and
instead of studying engineering I was studying philosophy. The world
was my oyster, and I was looking forward to the summer. I had been
accepted on an expedition to go to the North Pole, overland by dog
sled. I had already bought my boots. Nothing could stop me. And then
I got a cold, and the cold didn't go away, and I got sicker and sicker.
Over ten days it got to the point where I knew I was really sick.

I had never experienced being really sick before and I was afraid. I
didn't want to go to the doctor or the school nurse. I thought I'd bull
it through. And for about forty-eight hours I didn't sleep. I was in
agony. My neck was very stiff, my spine was aching, I had terrible pain.
And every step I took would radiate through me, up and down my
body. And if I lay down I was in even greater pain. So I spent two

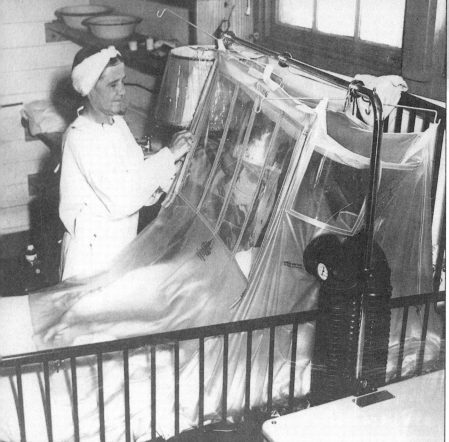

nights standing in the shower with hot water on my spine. And then I finally said, 'I have to go to the school nurse.' And she said, 'You have neuralgia. You've been lying in the grass reading books, I've seen you do that.' And she was right, I had been lying in the grass. So she gave me aspirin and I went away. And tried to get through my ordinary school routine. My parents were coming that night on a visit to the college. They had opposed my transferring, and it was going to be sort of a reconciliation. When my parents came in that night I rose from the couch to greet my father and I started to fall. I caught my knee, and he didn't notice. I managed to walk out to the car and then I walked across the yard with them to the infirmary, and it was the last time I walked. Those were the last steps I ever took.

The nurse said that she would call the doctor in the morning. My father insisted the doctor be called then. When he came I collapsed. I said, 'I don't know what it is, but I cannot stand the pain, you've got to do something.' So he had his black bag and he opened it and he pulled out a little tiny pill. And I said, 'No, I'm serious.' He said to just take it. Well, it turned out to be pure morphine and I went off to sleep. And woke in the morning and it was a beautiful sunny day, about six in the morning. The sun was streaming in the room and I lay there and watched as my legs became paralyzed. First the left leg moving up, and then the right leg moving down.

Talk about the acute phase, once you were in the hospital.

At the hospital I was put in quarantine in a little Quonset hut out back. The paralysis increased, climbed up my body over the next day and half. Until finally I was completely paralyzed, unable to move anything. My breathing became labored, and they put me in an oxygen tent. I thought the oxygen was failing because I wasn't getting anything. They sent for a surgeon from Philadelphia and he came out with police escort. And he did a tracheotomy. He cut my throat open as I was lying on the hospital bed because I was considered too far gone to move. And he couldn't use anaesthesia. I had so little breath reflex left, any anesthesia would have dampened the reflex. So I watched him do the surgery through the lenses on his eyeglasses, and I thought as soon as he cut it open that I would be able to breathe. But what he didn't have time to explain to me was that, once he cut it open, I would lose all sensation of any air coming through my nose or mouth. So he cut it open and all of a sudden I thought, 'I'm gone, I'm dead.' I was trying to tell him, and I couldn't move. I passed out and they called for volunteers and rushed me into the next room where the iron lung was. And I came to in the iron lung. And I was in the iron lung for about eight weeks.

Tell me about those eight weeks. You're not going to the North Pole.

No, I'm not. It brings back so many memories. I had a term paper I hadn't finished. And I kept thinking, 'Well, on Monday, I'll have to get out, I have to be well because I've got to get that term paper done.' In the iron lung, it wasn't a period of

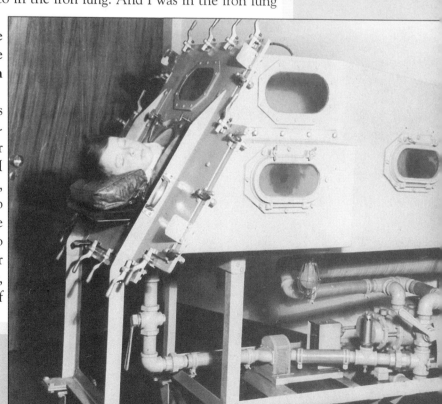

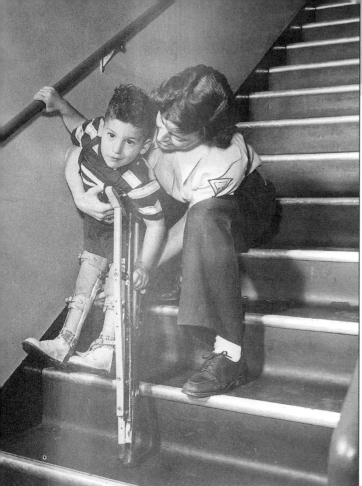

rest. There was so much to do, I mean I had two nurses a shift, six nurses a day, around the clock for three months. And we were all busy fighting to save my life. It's amazing the things that can go wrong in the human body. Everything went wrong. Everything. My bowels were impacted, my bladder didn't work. I had an infection in the bladder, I developed kidney stones. On top of everything else I had a tumor of the breast, which was unrelated. Those were a very difficult first couple of weeks, and I almost died several times. I had last rites, I said goodbye.

The acute phases passed, you got out of the iron lung. Talk about leaving the lung.

Being weaned from the iron lung is very difficult. It involved the therapist coming home from a cocktail party at night when I was asleep, stopping by, and turning off my iron lung to see how long I could breathe on my own. And so I'd wake up choking to death. And she began minute by minute and then doubling the time each day until the point where I could breathe on my own for two hours. Then I'd be taken out of the lung and put on a bed. It was terribly painful to be moved, and the kidney stones were beginning to cause problems, the infection was just awful. It was during the summer time and there was no air conditioning and the hot packs inside the iron lung were unbelievably annoying. And everybody, it seemed, was hurting me and one day I just lost it. And I've never done that before and I've never done it since. I just got hysterical, like people do on soap operas. And it had such an impact. Everybody was scared to death. I had my therapist, my doctor, my nurses, my family. There were so many people in the room always, and they all just stopped. And it was as though they were all hurting me, and they all stopped hurting me. I began to take some control again.

But polio is about losing control and rebuilding. Talk about rehabilitation.

I had worked very hard to separate from my parents, to strike out on my own, do it my way, and polio came like a bolt from heaven saying, 'You shouldn't have done that.' And I woke up and I'm back, as helpless as a baby, being nursed by my mother. I was determined that I would not live that way. Either I would live independent or I wouldn't live at all. I have found some old diaries that I wrote in the second year after polio. The first year I couldn't write because my hands didn't work, and that's what those diaries are about, how I am going to be independent. I remember in the diary I'd say, 'Mother pushed me today to Pennsylvania Avenue for a haircut. This was the first time I was out on the street. And as I was going down the street, a little girl passed me and she crossed herself as she passed me. And I thought, "Oh, she feels pity." And I wanted to go back to the hospital room right then. I wanted to hide.' And in the diary I wrote, 'She doesn't know how blessed I am to have a wonderful family and to have people who care.' But when I read the diary, what I remember instantly was my feeling with that little girl on the street.

You spent two years in the hospital. What did you do?

Oh, I ran the hospital by the end. It was run by Sisters of Charity, and I had a great big room. The Archbishop of Washington kept trying to get my room. He had a heart problem, but I lobbied with the sisters

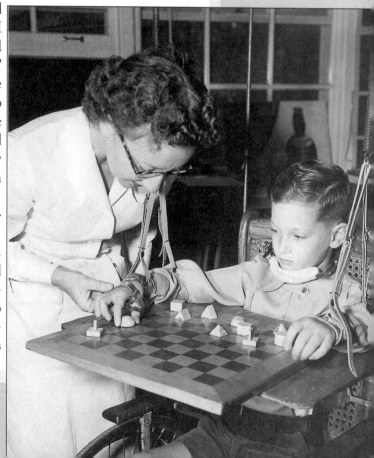

and I managed to keep it. And before he pulled rank, poor guy, he died and I kept my room. So I really hated to leave the hospital because I had a little world set up by then. I knew all the nurses, I knew all the doctors. And then I had to go to Warm Springs for rehabilitation. I didn't want to think of myself as crippled and I didn't want to associate with cripples. But I had to go; it was part of the independent business. So I flew down with my mother, and in those days airplanes weren't used to taking wheelchairs. They made the biggest production out of it, with fork lifts and people hauling and pulling. I have a photograph and I look really scared. And I certainly was really scared. But I got to Warm Springs and they put me in a room with three other people. When I first went in, there was this big tall guy lying down on a bed, doing the *New York Times* crossword puzzle. And he looked up and he said, 'What's a six-letter word meaning something-or-other.' And I just pulled it out of my head. And that was Lorenzo Milun. He and I have been close from that day to this. We talk at least two or three times a week. He lives on one end of the country, I live on the other. I made friends at Warm Springs that I have kept my entire life. Warm Springs changed my life totally. It showed me how I could live independently.

Tell me more about Warm Springs.

I still love Warm Springs. The dining room was a beautiful, sun-filled room, with white tablecloths, silver, and china. The staff didn't wear uniforms, but the waiters were dressed formally; the head waiter was in a dinner jacket. Seats were assigned. We had the best table. It was Lorenzo, me, Lumel, and Martha. And when I had to have surgery on my shoulders, we got my mother to come

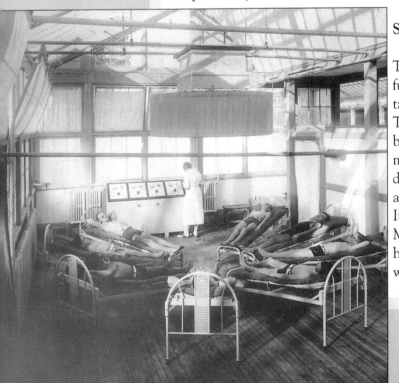

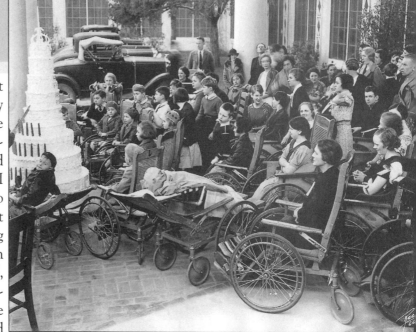

down and take my place at the table so that they wouldn't move someone who wasn't up to our standards. And after I had recovered from my surgery I couldn't get my mother to go home. I wanted that seat back, but she was having such a good time. Warm Springs is kind of isolated, and so we had a little society that was complete. We had love affairs, we had bridge tournaments, we had the latest movies. We had a newspaper with lots of gossip. And at the end of nine months I didn't want to go home.

You worked there, too.

The work was different from other rehab centers in that we concentrated on functional training. Learning how to get on and off toilets. Learning how to transfer from your bed to a wheelchair, from a wheelchair to a car. How to stand up, if you had the strength to do that. And we learned by watching others. Old polios would come back for checkups and there were a lot of polios who lived on the campus. And we would have functional training classes where—oh, they'd be so much fun 'cause they were so silly. You were having to learn these stupid things. I remember one class we were learning how to transfer from a car to a chair, and Lumel, who was such a beautiful girl, was transferring over and I was on the other side of the car watching her, and she just disappeared from sight. She'd missed. She hadn't hit the car, she hadn't hit the chair, she was just on the ground. And I remember seeing her just kind of disappear.

Did FDR still have a kind of presence at Warm Springs?

He had only been dead seven years by the time I got there. In fact my therapist had been one of his therapists. Whenever I met any-

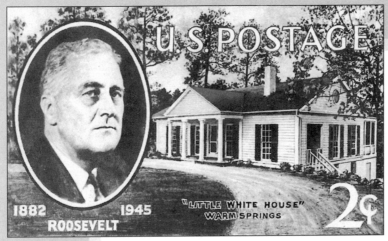

body who had known Roosevelt down there I always asked them, 'How did he handle his handicap?' Because I thought if he could do it, I could do it. I was a New Deal kid. And I'd been for FDR my whole life. I campaigned for him at the age of eight, and had been a page at the 1944 convention that renominated him. I joined the demonstration. In fact it was the Roosevelts who helped me into Warm Springs because in those days, with the epidemics, it was very hard to get in. And in terms of my rehabilitation he was sort of my role model. I think that was the role he played for most people down there. So Roosevelt just dominated Warm Springs.

At what point did you realize you weren't going to get better?

Remember I told you about my diary? Well, there is a one-line entry down in Warm Springs where it says, 'The Doctor told me that I will never walk again. There must be more to life.' And that's all I put in. I remember he was a nasty doctor. He was one of the doctors who was in charge of everything and everybody was afraid of him. Then he told me I'm never going to walk again. 'What you have is what you are going to have.' But he did say, 'Go talk to Fred Botts.' Botts was an old friend of Roosevelt's and together they had established Warm Springs. And Botts had about the same kind of paralysis as mine. I'm paralyzed from the shoulders down. But Botts was living an independent life and was the manager of the foundation down there. So I did go talk to Fred. And he helped me a lot. He showed me how he lived. And I began to think, 'That's not so bad. I can handle that. I've got to learn how to do it, but I can do that.'

Let's talk about your family and the effect polio had on them.

I've always figured that a disability is not an individual thing. It impacts not just me, but my family. I have a sister and I have a mother and father. I think the impact was as great on my sister as it was on me. She was just entering teenage years. She needed her mother and her mother was taken away from her because for two years my mother spent every day at the hospital, dedicated to keeping me alive. Everything was focused on me. There was an inner effect too, a subconscious effect that was more important. She's told me since, that she also had guilt feelings. That she feels maybe she should have been the one to have it. It's a very heavy burden. You know I think this crippled business is nine-tenths psychological and one-tenth physical. You can get up and down a curb by making a curb cut. But dealing with the psychological hurt is a lot more complicated.

How did polio make you different from other nineteen year olds?

Oh, when I almost died and I had all that pain, I learned a lot of things about life and what's important and what isn't. And the bitterness that goes with the nice. When I returned to college, it was as though I had been, say, upstairs in the house, and I knew what was upstairs. But my friends only lived on the ground floor and they didn't know there was a second floor. It was just an additional amount of knowledge. Everybody learns it, but usually it takes a lifetime. I learned it in a period of days.

Where did you go from there?

I had Roosevelt as a role model: he could do anything and so could I. And by God I did. I was one of those supercrips. I could do anything an able-bodied person could. I could do it faster, and so my career was fairly remarkable. I was the only person in a wheelchair at Oxford. I was the only person in a wheelchair on Capitol Hill for ten years. I

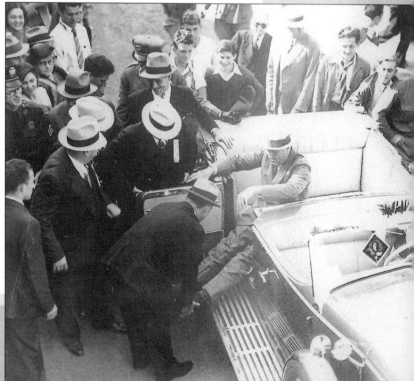

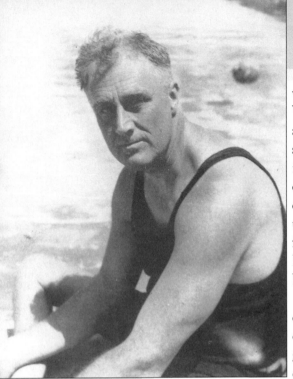

was the only person using a wheelchair at the White House during the Johnson era. I traveled around the world. I was charged by lions, stepped on by a hippopotamus. Rode a dogsled in Alaska. But I had no life. I confused my career with my life. I confused proving myself to others with having a life of my own. And I was using all my energy, I see now, to keep up this facade of being happy, carefree, efficient, intelligent, successful. And there was nothing behind it.

And then one day, I collapsed. I had a breakdown. Physically and mentally. And the way it came to me was through this big blackbird. I was giving a speech up in Alaska, and in the middle of the speech, all of a sudden I heard this huge bird up there, and it flapped its wings. It was as real as anything. And when I collapsed, that big blackbird was sitting on my shoulder. He sat on my shoulder for several days. I couldn't move. I couldn't transfer. I couldn't function. I couldn't eat. I now know it was the beginning of a great situational depression. I had never dealt with this catastrophe that had hit me when I was nineteen. I'd never even thought about it. I mean, I had kept myself from thinking and from feeling. I hadn't had a dream in twenty years. I just had erased my emotional life. I killed it. And it all came upon me like gangbusters. All the grief, all the hurt, all the might-have-beens, all the self-pity, everything. And it incapacitated me. I had to work to get out of that depression for several years. But in the process I learned so much about myself. I learned who I am and how my disability is me and that's who I am, and to get on. And my life has been incomparably better as a result.

What happened to the blackbird?

The blackbird flew away.

Let's talk about FDR and how polio affected him.

FDR was a beautiful construction. Who was it, Jung, the great psychiatrist, who said FDR must have been analyzed by God? He had such a buoyancy, he had such cheer, he had such warmth that people were attracted to him, people loved him. He had a giant head. He used that head to project his feelings. He had a long cigarette holder that he'd cock up and that would make everybody feel good. He had the old beat-up campaign hat that he wore during the four campaigns and made him look as comfortable as an old shoe. He had that great military cape that he wore, especially during wartime. He had the glasses like Woodrow Wilson. These were all images that he learned to use and project, and he had learned how to do that because he was a paraplegic. He was in a wheelchair. He could not stand up and stalk around a room or work a cocktail party and press the flesh. He had to draw people to him.

People say they remember FDR walking across the room.

Yes. People just weren't aware of his disability, even when they observed it. In the 1932 campaign, my mother heard Roosevelt speak from the balcony of the Grand Palace Hotel in Denver. She couldn't have been more than twenty feet away from him, and she said she did not remember that he had any trouble getting to the podium at all. It was a deception that was very cleverly arranged, but the people loved him so and wanted to see him as all-powerful. And they just didn't perceive their president as being in any way disabled. He always said, 'I had polio, I was crippled, but I'm a cured cripple now. I may have a limp, but that's all.'

There are only two known photographs of Roosevelt using a wheelchair, and yet he was in a wheelchair most of the day. As I say in my book, it was FDR's splendid deception. It was a way of keeping the public from

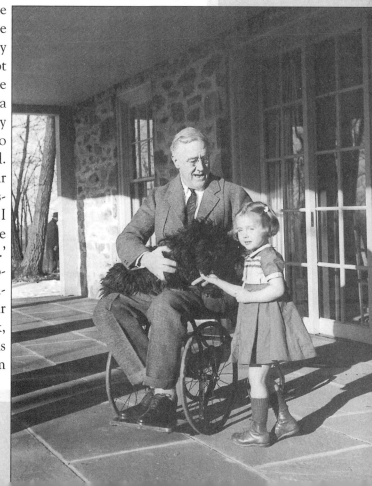

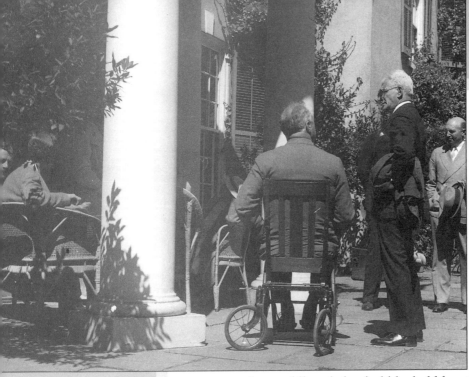

dwelling on the fact that he was incapacitated. I mean, these were the days when disabled people were considered impolite. They were not supposed to be seen in public. They were supposed to be invalids, kept upstairs in the bedroom with the shades drawn. And Franklin Roosevelt was out in the middle of the hubble bubble of politics. If he had appeared before the public as a paraplegic, that's what the public would have remembered. He had a campaign to win. He had achievements to give the American people. So the deception was a way of allowing him to provide the leadership without making disability an issue.

How do you think polio changed FDR?

His family, especially the Republican side of his family, had always considered him to be a lightweight. They called him the featherduster. They didn't expect him to amount to much. And indeed people have said that he was a playboy, living on his mother's money until he got polio. Polio changed him. He had had a life of unparalleled success until then. He was an only son and his mother adored him, showered him with attention. He had always been given anything he wanted. And then he got polio. Polio was the only thing that he had ever confronted that he couldn't beat. He had decided, 'I'm going to lick this, I'm going to walk again.' And seven years of his life were devoted entirely to rehabilitation. And he didn't win. He was no more rehabilitated at the end of seven years than he was at the beginning.

He did learn some tricks in functional training at Warm Springs. He learned how to give the appearance of standing and walking. He wore long leg braces, and he always wore black trousers, black socks, black shoes, and always painted the braces black so they didn't stand out. Sometimes he wore a body brace that would hitch to the leg braces to give him stability, because he would buckle at the hips when he stood without that brace. And he could stand without the pelvic band, as it was called, but if there was a slight breeze or a jostle, he'd go. He could stand holding on to a podium. He could stand with crutches. He developed a technique with his sons. They were four strong, strapping young men, and they took arm training, strengthening their arms so that they had the power of a parallel bar. And he would lean on the arm of a son to hitch this side, and he would use a cane with his other arm. And by shifting all his weight from one side to the other he was able to kind of toddle. It was dangerous. His therapist told someone that she could never watch Roosevelt in a newsreel or in public without holding her breath, she was so afraid he might fall.

FDR was different at Warm Springs.

Yes, he was alive as a person. When he was president, he was always on stage, always performing, always the center of attention. And he never talked about how he felt about being paralyzed. He never talked to his mother, by her testimony, or his wife, or his children. And this was like an emotional wall between him and the ones who were closest and who loved him so much. At Warm Springs, perhaps more than

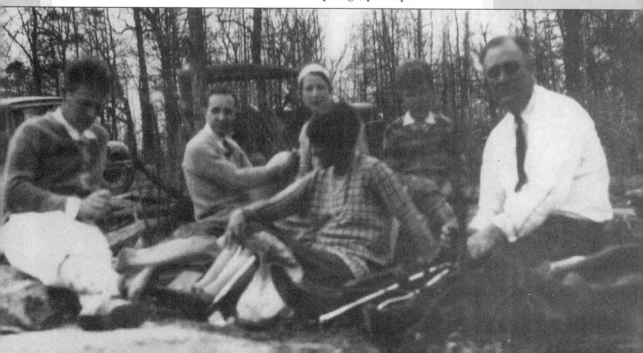

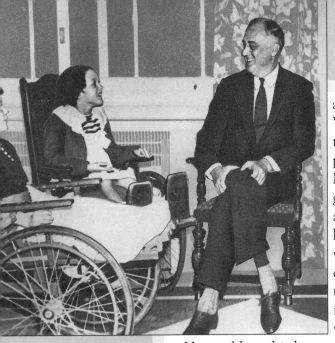

anywhere else, he was a human being. The Warm Springs foundation was several thousand acres entirely fenced in, patrolled around its perimeter by the Marine Corps. So that once the President got inside the foundation, he could do anything he wanted. And he never wore his braces at Warm Springs. He used his wheelchair, he swam in the pool with the other polios, he went around to the wards, talked to everybody. He played bridge up in Georgia Hall with the patients. He went to Chapel.

He would put his braces on at Chapel to walk in for the newsreel cameras, and everyday in the afternoon he'd get in his little car and drive down to the gate and meet the reporters and have an impromptu press conference with them. But other than that, in Warm Springs he was a polio with other polios and was very comfortable. He was never bothered about being crippled. He would drive around Warm Springs with the top down on his little Model A Ford coupe and stop and chat with neighbors. Sometimes he'd go and pay a call on someone and if he didn't have his wheelchair with him he'd bounce to the ground on his butt, and, sort of bounce up the walk into the house. He was very comfortable with himself that way.

In the age and society Roosevelt lived in, people didn't talk about unpleasant things. People lived life on the tea-party level. And it worked very well for Roosevelt, in the sense that he was able to function very successfully. After all, he was the greatest president of the twentieth century. But his emotional life was shriven. It was virtually non-existent. He said once when he met Orson Welles, 'Orson, you and I are the two best actors in America.' And he was right, you know. And that's not a good way to live. Denial plays a useful role but there comes a time when it becomes worse than a deception. It becomes an obstruction between you and leading a life of meaning and communication with your loved ones.

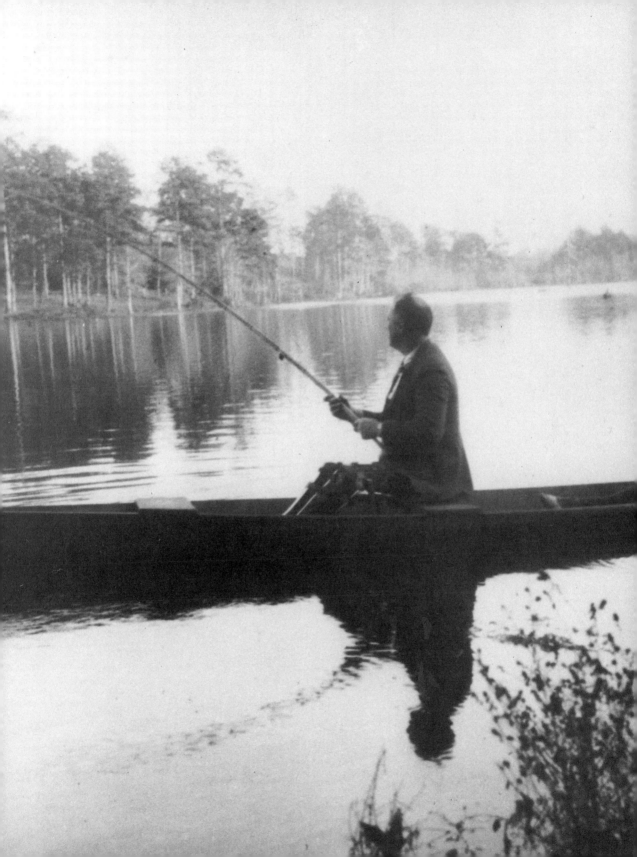

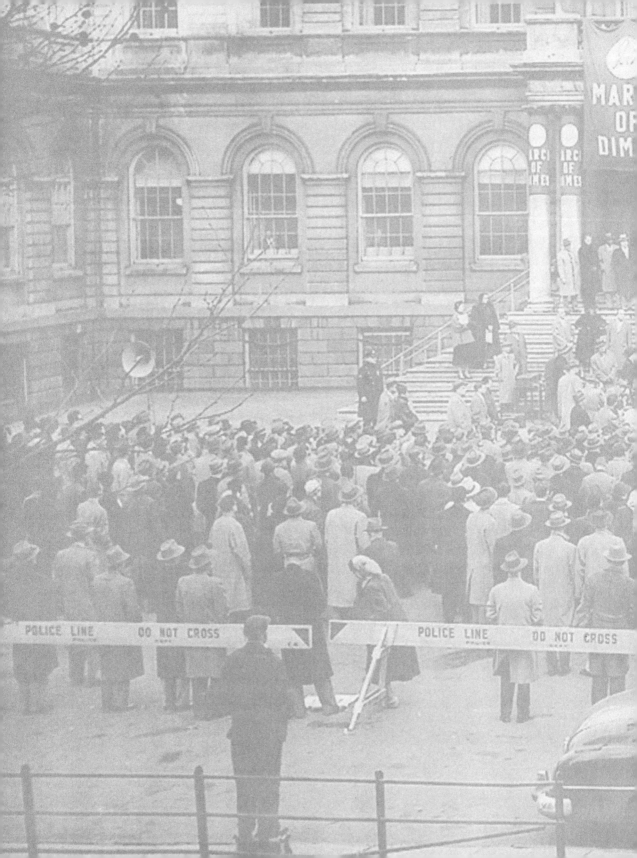

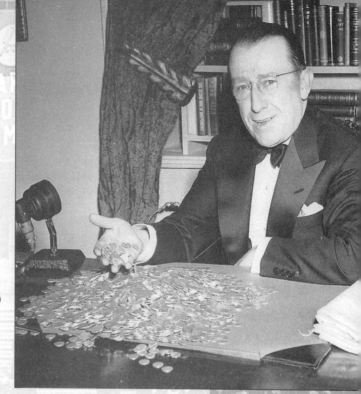

Chapter 3

Politics, Hollywood, and Money

The volunteers were really the homemakers. They came from almost everywhere because everybody felt an excitement about the prospect of doing something for this terrible problem. . . . The March of Dimes had affiliations with PTAs, with business and professional women, all kinds of library clubs, all kinds of organizations of women. Most of the men were already tied to the Rotary Club or Kiwanis Club or the Junior Chamber of Commerce, all kinds of organizations of men that had been involved in the war effort so they were already conditioned to do civic work. This brought the mothers into the picture. So you had whole families that were committed, and that was the way things were done in the 1950s.

—Charles Massey,
former president of the March of Dimes

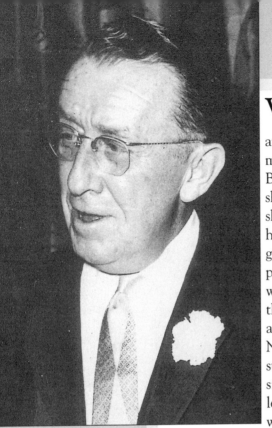

When Franklin Roosevelt left Warm Springs in 1928 to campaign for Governor of New York and then for the presidency in 1932, he handed the management of the therapy center to his law partner, Basil O'Connor. The two men had joined forces shortly after Roosevelt's paralysis, and their partnership was a study in opposites. Roosevelt was tall and handsome, heir to a respectable fortune and a distinguished name. Basil O'Connor was the small, unprepossessing, ambitious son of Irish immigrants, a man who had worked his way through college by playing the fiddle at student parties. When O'Connor approached the convalescing former Secretary of the Navy to join his Wall Street law firm, offering a steady income with no effort in exchange for the simple privilege of putting Roosevelt's name on his letterhead, he had no idea that his new partner would soon add polio to the firm's list of clients.

In later years, after he had devoted most of his life to conquering polio, Basil O'Connor told interviewer Richard Carter of his reluctant entry into the polio cause. "In 1928 [Roosevelt] ups and becomes Governor of New York and nonchalantly says to me, 'Take over Warm Springs, old fella: you're in.' I tell you, I had no desire to be 'in.' I was never a public do-gooder and had no aspirations of that kind. But I started enjoying it. Like Andrew Jackson at the Battle of New Orleans, I found myself up to my rump in blood and loving it."

O'Connor knew that Roosevelt could not pay for the care of the many polio survivors who flocked to Warm Springs in his wake, hoping for a cure that had eluded the handsome politician. New sources of funding would have to be found if Warm Springs was to continue as a center for polio rehabilitation. In 1926, O'Connor had helped Roosevelt avoid financial ruin by making the resort into a nonprofit foundation, raising money from wealthy patients, their families, and friends. Soon, however, it became clear that even this would not be enough. While most people saw the election of 1932 as a ray of light breaking through the darkness of the Depression, Basil O'Connor recognized Roosevelt's election to the White House as the solution to the polio funding problem. He began to do nothing less than use the prestige of the presidency to serve his new cause.

Soon the Georgia Warm Springs Foundation was joined by the National Foundation for Infantile Paralysis. Like its name, the mission of the new foundation was national, not local. So was its fundraising. The first campaign was a series of annual balls, pegged to Roosevelt's birthday at the end of January and promoted with the slogan, "dance so that others may walk." In the first year, 1935, six thousand "President's Birthday Balls" raised almost eight hundred thousand dollars, ten times what O'Connor had anticipated. The money was used for patient care at Warm Springs and to finance research into the cause and prevention of polio.

By 1938, Roosevelt had been president for six years. The birthday balls had run their course, bringing in less money each year. Epidemics continued, however, and the costs of caring for polio patients did not decrease. Nor did the price of doing research to improve that care or find a way of stopping the rising toll of epidemics. The National Foundation had pledged to support the needs of polio patients, but it needed a fresh approach to keep that promise.

The new direction for the National Foundation came from a former vaudeville star who had found even greater fame on the radio, but who had never forgotten the way the Democratic Party had watched out for the poor immigrants in his child-

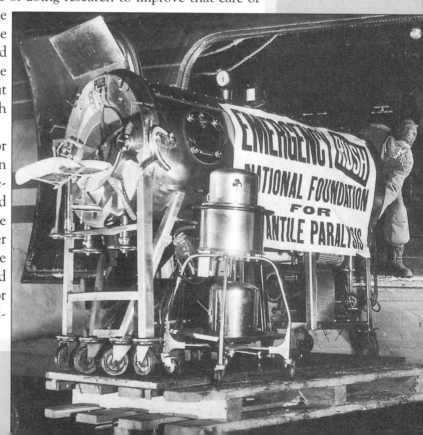

hood neighborhood on New York's Lower East Side. Eddie Cantor, one of the country's most popular entertainers, was already a fundraiser for both the Democratic Party and the President's Birthday Balls. Now he suggested a new sort of charity appeal, for which he coined the name "The March Of Dimes," a wordplay on the popular contemporary newsreel series "The March Of Time." It was democratic with a small *d*, an appeal that went out across the nation, calling on every citizen to work for the common good. You did not have to be a millionaire or a regular on the charity-ball circuit to join the fight against polio. Anyone could give a dime.

Roosevelt had many supporters in Hollywood, and the National Foundation had professional publicists and campaign directors as talented and sophisticated as the actors who volunteered to spread the

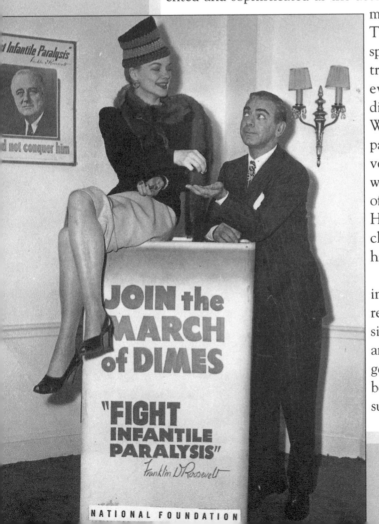

message of the March of Dimes. Through posters and leaflets, radio spots and movie shorts, the country's most popular performers told everyone to send their dimes directly to the White House in Washington. Once again, the campaign was keyed to President Roosevelt's birthday. The public response was fast and enthusiastic. A deluge of silver coins flooded the White House mail room. From then on, charity and show business went hand in hand in the war on polio.

When the March of Dimes began in 1938, the United States was still recovering from the Great Depression. Few people had medical insurance, and the federal "safety net" of government programs was still being woven. Nor was there any substantial federal support for med-

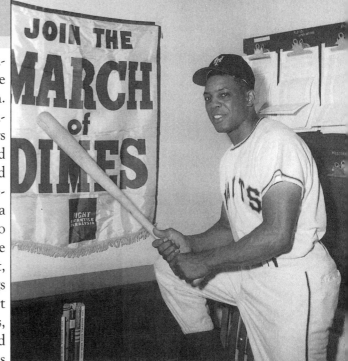

ical research on polio, either for prevention or after-care. Into this considerable void stepped the National Foundation. With the money raised by local foundation chapters, the national headquarters financed the care of old patients and new, gave scholarships to nurses and doctors who needed training in the specific care of polio patients, and funded a broad spectrum of laboratory research to increase fundamental knowledge of the disease. Equipment had to be bought, from splints and crutches to iron lungs and the large trucks it took to transport them to epidemic areas. Doctors, nurses, and physical therapists had to be trained in the latest methods, and publications had to be issued, outlining preferred treatment techniques. The costs of all this were enormous, and the number of people needing help mounted with each new polio epidemic.

On top of the costs of patient care, medical training, and research, there came the costs of keeping the public committed to the fight against polio. As the expenses mounted, so did the intensity of the fundraising campaigns. Any means, even blatant fear-mongering, was deemed acceptable if it led to the end of polio. Mickey Mouse led a marching band in a chorus of "Hi ho, hi ho, we'll lick that polio." Dime by dime and dollar by dollar, they raised the funds to support the research that would fulfill O'Connor's dream and "lick polio in my lifetime."

Over the years, the speakers changed but the campaign remained the same. Top stars from Mickey Rooney to Elvis Presley filmed fundraising appeals that aired in movie theaters, on radio, and later on television. They spoke as themselves, the gods and goddesses of Hollywood stepping down from their pedestals to reveal that they, too, feared polio and yearned for ways to help the cause. Greer Garson invited the audience

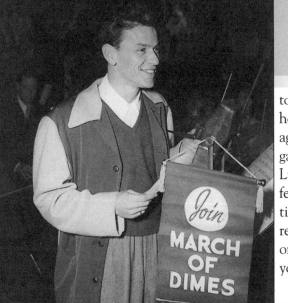

to come with her to Hickory, North Carolina, to see how bravely the citizens had marshaled their forces against polio—and how essential the money they gave to the March of Dimes had been. Helen Hayes, Lucille Ball, and Zsa Zsa Gabor all confided their fears, mother to mother, and begged for contributions. They were actresses, but the emotion was real; Hayes' daughter had died of polio, and everyone knew that no amount of fame could protect your family from the dreaded infection.

The campaigns might be slick, but the cause retained its popular support because it spoke to every level of American society. This was a grass-roots organization with a national mission, operating without any involvement from the federal government. From nationwide campaigns to community programs, the National Foundation controlled its own agenda, from designing posters and armbands to ordering iron lungs, educating nurses, and funding research. Decisions came from 120 Broadway, the same Wall Street address where O'Connor still maintained his law firm, but much of the work of collecting money and distributing information was done by community volunteers in local chapters that sprang up across the country.

World War II brought another crisis, and another change, to the war on polio. O'Connor had feared that the demands of war—and the campaigns to sell war bonds—would rob support from the polio cause. Instead, contributions rose. Women were enlisted to take the place of the male fundraisers who had gone to war, and a new emphasis on polio as a family issue dominated the March of Dimes campaigns. Here on the home front, women were reminded, we must protect our children. While

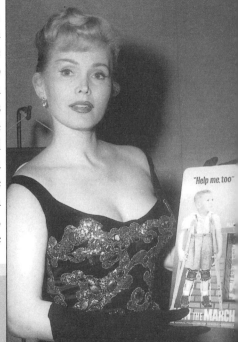

"Help me, too"

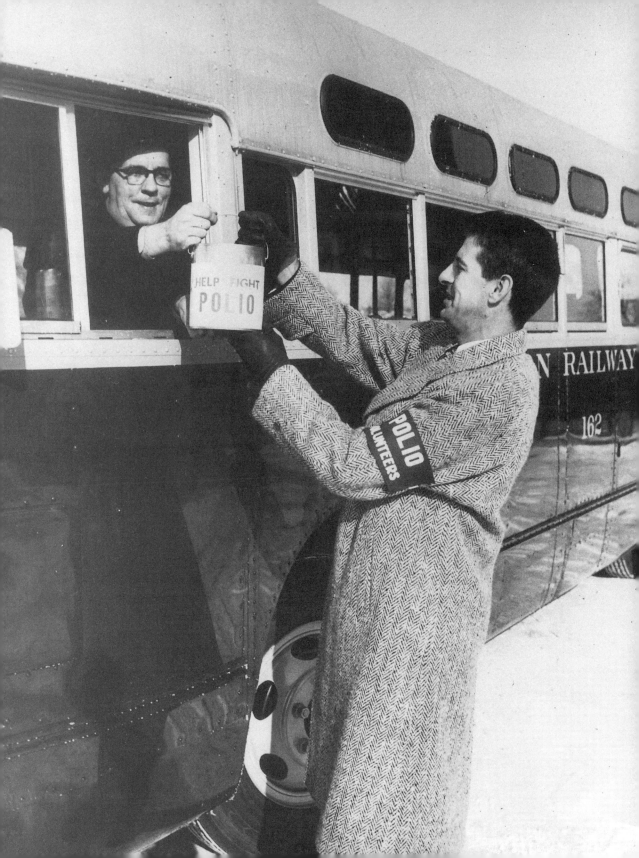

you are away, soldiers were told, the National Foundation stands ready to take care of your family. As ever, Franklin Roosevelt remained honorary president of the National Foundation—his name on the letterhead meant as much now as it had when O'Connor had first asked him to be his legal partner.

Starting in 1946, the National Foundation introduced another fundraising innovation, the Poster Child. Along with the annual selection of a national Poster Child, announced with much fanfare and featured in the publicity for that year's March of Dimes campaign, there were also regional and local "poster children." Boys and girls, black and white, affected in visibly different ways by the polio virus, represented a juvenile spectrum of polio survivors. With all their differences, however, all the poster children embodied youthful health and promise—except for the metal braces that encased their legs, the crutches that enabled them to walk, the slings that held their helpless arms in place, or the braces that supported their heads.

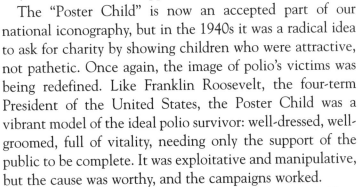

The "Poster Child" is now an accepted part of our national iconography, but in the 1940s it was a radical idea to ask for charity by showing children who were attractive, not pathetic. Once again, the image of polio's victims was being redefined. Like Franklin Roosevelt, the four-term President of the United States, the Poster Child was a vibrant model of the ideal polio survivor: well-dressed, well-groomed, full of vitality, needing only the support of the public to be complete. It was exploitative and manipulative, but the cause was worthy, and the campaigns worked.

People who were closest to the realities of life after polio—children whose able-bodied friends had abandoned them, parents who struggled to care for their baby in an iron lung, hopefuls who came to Warm Springs but never did find a cure—sometimes grew cynical about the up-beat message of the March of Dimes campaigns. They might complain about the unreal, impossible perfection of the poster child image. But they would also be grateful for the difficult, expensive treatment that was paid for with money raised by the inspiring, optimistic, wallet-opening image of the poster child.

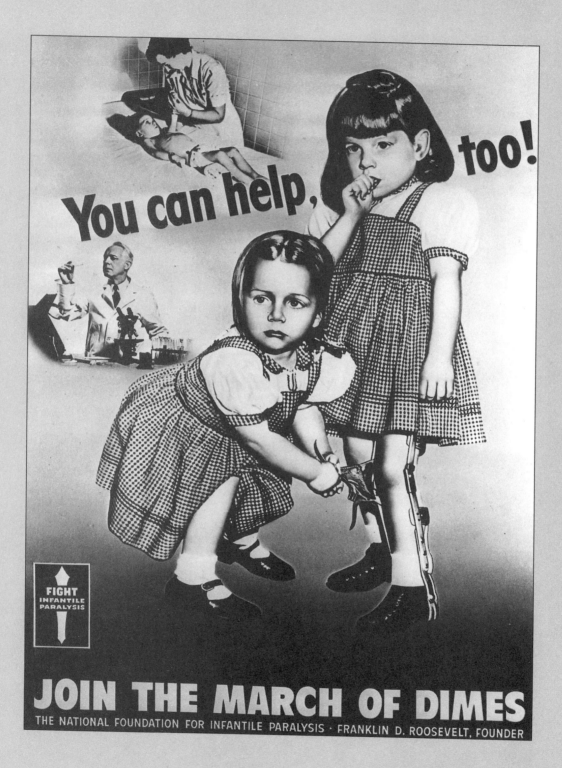

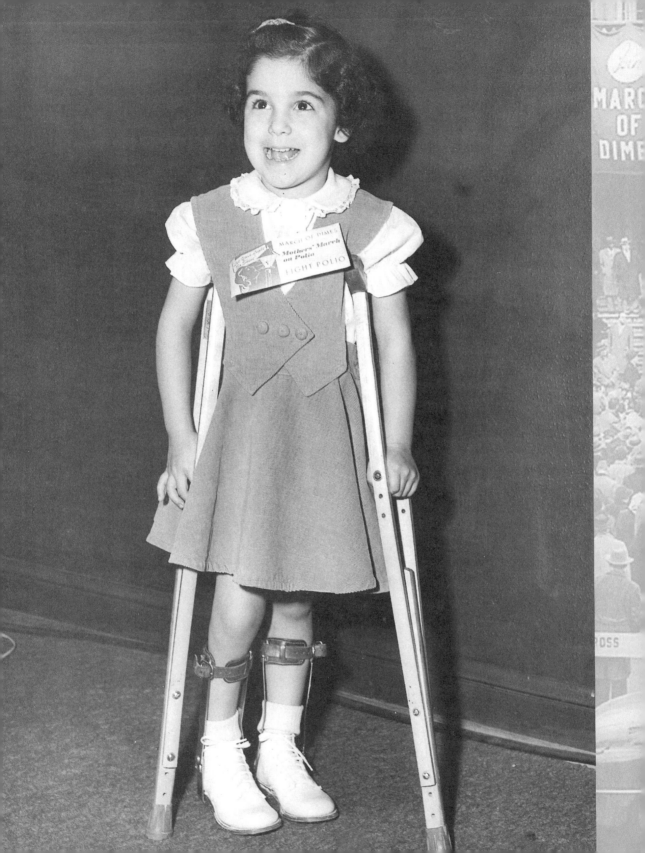

Voices
Carol Boyer

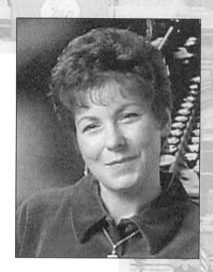

Carol Boyer was three years old in 1952 when she contracted polio. She became a poster child for the March of Dimes for the District of Columbia. She was photographed with movie stars and with then-Vice President Richard Nixon.

How old were you when you had the first signs of polio?

I was three years old. It was 1952. I remember I was sleeping, and I needed to get up to go to the bathroom and I fell out of my bed. When I went to put my legs over the side of the bed, I couldn't get up, I just fell. I couldn't understand what was wrong. I remember crawling to my parents' bed. I don't even know whether I made it to the bathroom. But I remember crawling down the hallway up to their bed and told my mom that something was wrong. I couldn't walk. That was when I first discovered something was going wrong in my body.

I was taken to Children's Hospital [in Washington, D.C.], and they first diagnosed me as having meningitis. I don't really remember all the tests that were being done to me, but I do remember being left alone without my mom quite a bit. It took them a few days before they realized what I really had was what they called infantile paralysis.

Tell me what you remember about your mom's leaving?

They put you in a white hospital bed with the bars up. It was crib-like. At three years old they were afraid you were going to fall out. And I remember the very small windows next to my bed that I could look out. They did let my mom stay with me quite a few nights, but eventually she had my brother to take care of, she couldn't stay with me forever. It was what psychologists call separation anxiety, and I remember it was awful being left alone without my mom. I just cried and cried

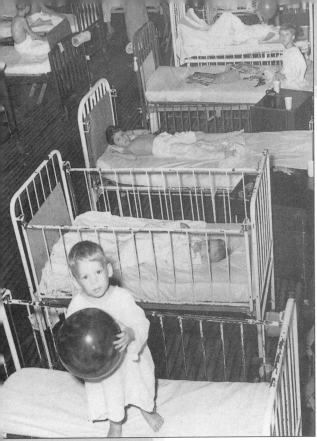

and cried. I remember hearing children crying. And I know I was there for quite some time, from right before Thanksgiving until May, about six months.

What else do you remember from that time?

I do remember seeing a few people in iron lungs—men and women, and that was very very scary to me, to see people that had to be flat on their backs, only their heads stuck out of this big, white, cylindrical machine. I thought they didn't have bodies. I was afraid of what was happening to these people. I thought how hard this is for people to have to look at their friends and family through a mirror above their face. And I just thought that was the most awful thing. I used to have nightmares, and they lasted for quite some time, way up until probably my preteens. I used to have this nightmare in which there were two very short men with long white coats down in my parents' basement, and they were going to put me in this ringer-type of machine, like the old washing machines, and mangle up my legs. And I would scream. I didn't have the nightmares after I was a teen, but it never dawned on me 'til I was older that it had to be the iron lung.

How did you get your picture on a poster?

I really don't know how I was selected. I was at Children's Hospital, which was one of the foremost polio research and treatment places in the United States. And I was selected to be the District of Columbia poster child for the March of Dimes campaign. And all of a sudden I was going on photo shoots. The dress in the picture was green. Kelly green. I remember I felt very special. My mother told me we were going to a special fundraiser for the March of Dimes. We traveled all around the Washington area, and I just remember my mother telling me there's all these people that are going to be there that are contributing money to the March of Dimes and they want to meet you. It was a big apartment complex on Connecticut Avenue, and they had me on a coffee table. And it was nice, I guess, being the center of attention. And it has probably shaped my life because you're put in the limelight, you have all these people asking you questions and wondering who you are, asking where you go to school or what you do with your time. It was fun but it also made you feel like you have to look perfect, you have to be this, you have to be that, and make sure you have courteous manners and things of the sort.

My mother explained to me one day that there was going to be a very special photo shoot that was going to be happening, and it would be with the President. Or if he couldn't show up, the Vice President would show up. And I remember her telling me over and over again so I wouldn't make a mistake because I was so young. 'The President is bald, and the Vice President has dark hair.' And I must have been told that over and over again so I wouldn't say, 'Thank you, Mr. Vice President' to the President. And lo and behold, Vice President Nixon was

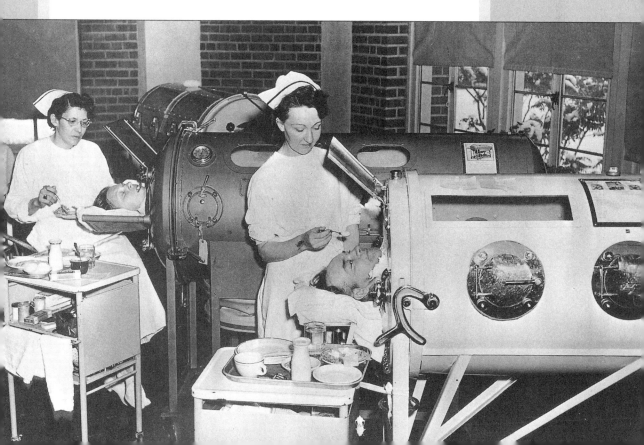

the one that did show up, and I did know that it was the Vice President. You know, you hear 'Vice President Nixon' on the TV and the radio, so I knew that was someone important coming to see me. They had another little girl with me, and a congressman was there, and a newsreel was made. About a month later we got a call from my mother's relatives in New York who happened to be watching a movie in the theater and called up very excited saying that they saw Carol at the movies.

One of the photo shoots had Patricia Crowley, an actress who was a starlet then. I remember vividly, she was pouring a bunch of dimes into my skirt. She was sitting down on top of some high piece of furniture and the dimes were pouring in. I remember a lot of my photos were with women that were working for the March of Dimes, with their daughters spelling out 'Mother's March' all in dimes on a beautiful carpet. So I did realize that I had something to do with helping people with polio just like myself.

What happened at school after all the attention and the polio?

Kids teased me, they liked to play with my crutches. Up until the

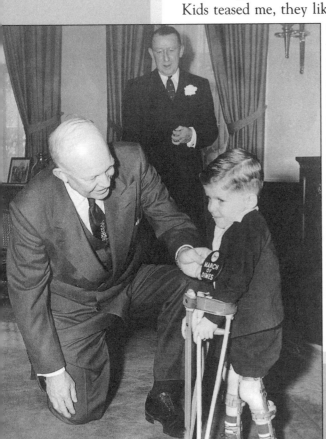

time I was about twelve years old I walked with crutches, I had braces on both of my legs. I had to wear a corset as I got a little older, with steel stays in them around my back 'cause I had a swayback. I corrected that with exercising. But I was uncomfortable. Then I had surgery, and I was one of those success stories that the orthopedic surgeons like to take to their conferences and show colleagues their great success with a particular patient. So I didn't have the crutches as I got past thirteen years old. But kids would copy limping like me. They'd walk in front of me. I was always picked last in kickball games. Who wanted me on their team? I couldn't run fast, I couldn't kick with both of my legs.

Ardean Martin

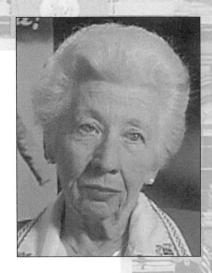

Ardean Martin was the General Chairman of the Mothers March on Polio for San Diego County in 1951. In 1955, she was on hand at Lindbergh Field in San Diego when the first shipment of the Salk vaccine was delivered for distribution.

How did you get involved with raising money to fight polio?

The very first time I ever heard of a march or a door-to-door collection, I was at a dinner at which one of the speakers was Basil O'Connor, a personal friend of President Roosevelt. I was a director of health for the PTA of San Diego County. At that time we were all very frightened because we had an epidemic of polio in San Diego County, more cases than there had ever been before. And, of course, I had a son at that time who was six years old. So I went to the March of Dimes office, and we organized parent and teacher groups from all over. We explained to them that we were going to do the Mother's March on Polio and do everything we could to raise money for this Salk vaccine that we had briefly heard about. The very first one was held about the first of February in 1951. There were probably eight or nine hundred people that went out and the theme was this: If you want to contribute toward fighting polio, turn on your porchlight at seven o'clock, and those were the only places that were called upon. I stayed at the March of Dimes headquarters to take phone calls from people who wanted to tell us where they lived and that nobody called on them. Many children accompanied their parents. Maybe they could only give a nickel or a dime, but every dime counted. We were working toward one goal, to eliminate polio. I made some wonderful, wonderful friends through the Mother's March that I kept all these years. It just seemed that everyone was grateful they had a part in it. It's a feeling of self-satisfaction and love.

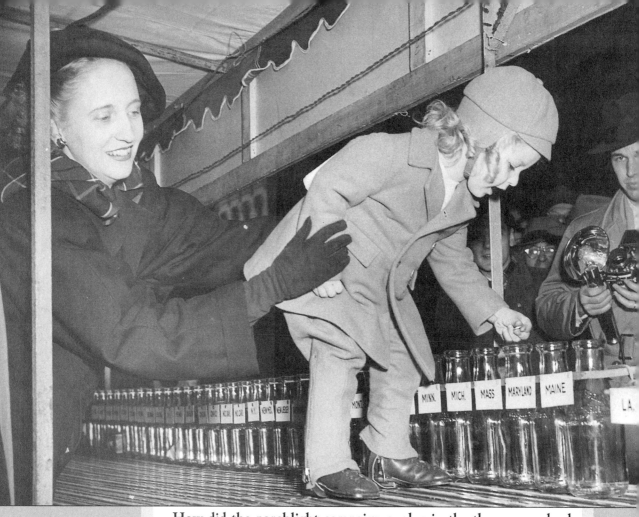

How did the porchlight campaign evolve in the three years leading up to the vaccine?

The more people heard there would be a vaccine it seemed like [the easier it was to raise money]. The last year, when we had reports that they were working on it, we raised more money and had more people going door-to-door than ever before. We just had no problem that year. In fact calls were made, 'Can I march?' I don't think there was a house that was missed in San Diego County. The church bells were ringing, several fire stations would blow their horns to say that this was the hour, seven o'clock, time to turn on your porchlight. One man told me he just sat in his car and blew the horn so people would know. I was coordinating it from San Francisco to San Diego and on this particular night porchlights went on from one end of California to the other.

Tell me what you remember when it was announced on April 12 that the Salk vaccine was a success.

Well, that's a day I shall never, never forget. The day that you read in the papers, 'We don't have to worry about polio, the vaccine has proven successful,' was a great highlight in my life. I was among those who went to Lindbergh Field when they flew the first box of Salk vaccine into San Diego, and I could remember the director of health for San Diego saying, 'Here, you take it, you deserve it. You've done more for this than anybody.' And I stood there with the tears running down my cheeks and I just said, 'Thank you, God. Thank you.'

What did you think was going to happen, now that you had this vaccine?

I felt that it was going to take time, it wasn't going to be an overnight success. We set up stations in different areas and the school nurses cooperated with us under the supervision of a doctor in each area. We had certain ages, like five to nine, that received the shots first, and then the older ones. I can remember in my particular area that people were lined up around the block, and of course the children screamed and yelled. I remember when my son got the shot, I thought, 'This is the day that I walked for.'

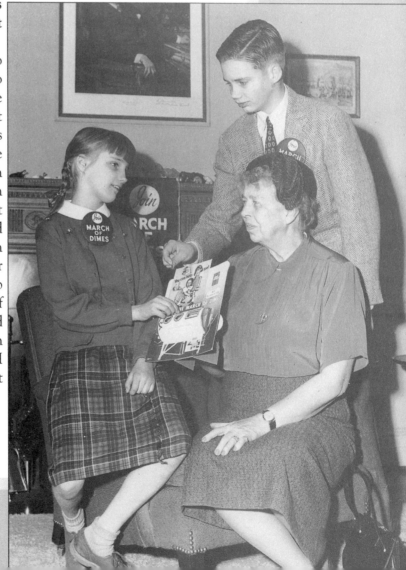

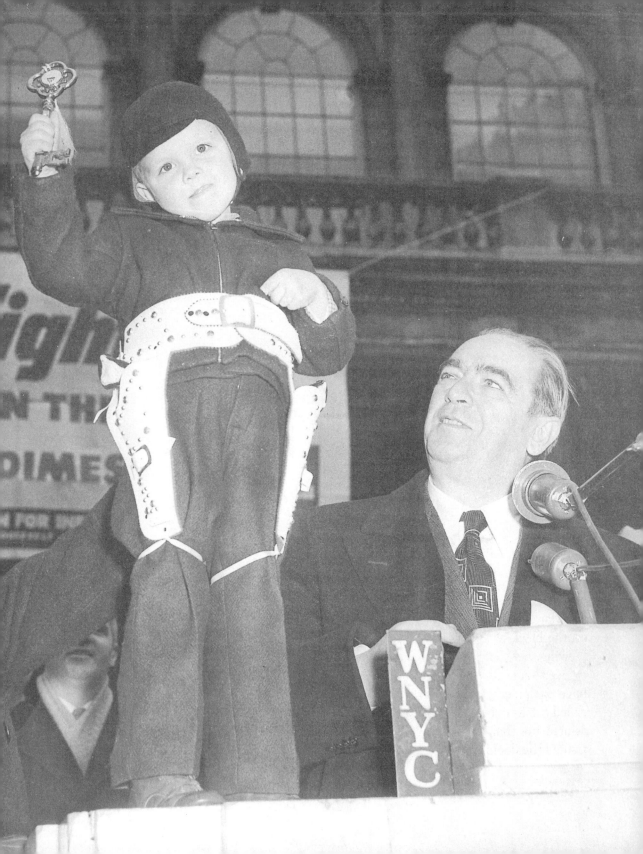

Charles Massey

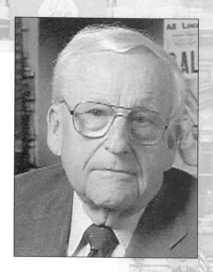

Charles Massey's first job with the March of Dimes was in 1948, organizing local chapters in Arkansas, Kentucky, and Georgia. He continued his career with the March of Dimes and ultimately became its president from 1978 to 1989.

Paint a picture of what the Arkansas epidemic was like.

I might want to start in 1948. My first job with the March of Dimes was to set up a chapter structure in Arkansas. My job was to start traveling the state, meet with groups of volunteers or potential volunteers, and set up chapters for all seventy-five counties. I finished that job in about one year. So in the middle of 1949, I was feeling pretty good about myself and felt this job had been done—I can go do something else. All of a sudden I receive a phone call from University Hospital, which was the only hospital in the state that would accept polio patients at that time. They said they had just heard that a polio case was coming in from the north part of the state. They were kind of giving me an alert, wondering if this was the beginning of an epidemic, or just a single case. Before the day was out, we had several other phone calls. And before two days had gone by all six of the isolation beds at the hospital had been filled. The doctor in charge there called me and said, 'I understand the March of Dimes is responsible for polio.' And so, I was the new kid on the block and I really didn't realize the potential problem that was brewing. So I said, 'Yes, I'm responsible.' And he said, 'Well, I'm going to need some help. We only have limited space here and we have to have equipment, nurses and doctors, and iron lungs, you name it.' So I called the March of Dimes headquarters office with this news, and they assured me that whatever we needed we would get. Based on that I assured the doctor that we would take care of this.

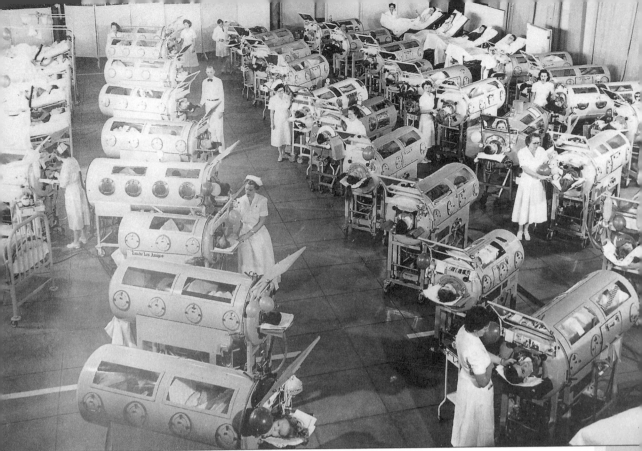

But the cases kept coming in from all over the state. What we did first was to take over the nursing residence at the University Hospital and move the nurses out and set up a respirator center there. There were about thirty respirators that were set up initially. But that was just a temporary measure, because even with the maximum capacity of the University Hospital, they could not take the cases as they were coming in. We had to concentrate on opening up space in the other hospitals. Now, the March of Dimes, faced with the same problem a few years earlier in North Carolina, had set up a sort of Army type of hospital arrangement in Hickory, North Carolina. And they did not want to go through that again. My job, they told me, was to see that this problem was dealt with without creating emergency facilities. That meant that I had to go the Arkansas Baptist Hospital and the St. Vincent Hospital and talk to the administration about relaxing their ban on polio cases. The whole concern they had was one growing out of fear. Everybody was afraid of polio and afraid of contagion in the hospital. So we went through a little tug-of-war for several days, while they resisted accepting these patients. And the patients were still coming into the University Hospital. What I did was to call the newspapers in and to take some pictures of the situation at University Hospital. Some of the patients were actually in the hall at that point. And a few days after that, the administrator of Baptist Hospital called and said he had changed his mind. He would accept the patients if we could provide the equipment. He would give over the chapel as a polio ward if we could equip it. So I said, 'Fine, we could do that.' And I was hoping I was right. I called the New York office and they assured me that everything would be taken care of. So, in a matter of three days, nurses were arriving in Little Rock, physical therapists were arriving, and equipment was arriving. Some of the beds actually were flown in from Hickory, North Carolina, where they had been stored. And in one week we had a working polio ward in Baptist Hospital.

What was the tenor of the media during that epidemic?

Well, they were trying to express their civic concern for this problem: Cases were being admitted to hospitals in other states, why can't we admit them here in Arkansas? They were appealing to the conscience of the hospital's administration, and they were dramatizing the plight of the University Hospital, which, by law, had to take the patients. They were in effect creating a motivation on the part of the hospitals to overcome the fear of polio. What it really amounted to was that the fear of doing nothing was made greater than the fear of polio. And so, shortly after the Baptist Hospital made the announcement, Sister Margaret Louise from St. Vincent's called me to say that she felt patients in St. Vincent's ought to receive their care at her hospital. She

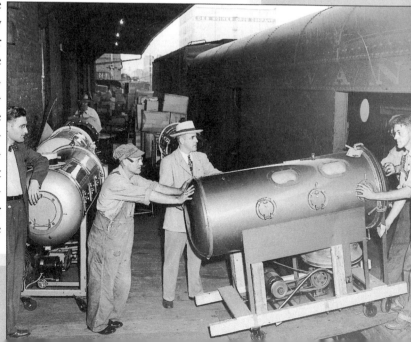

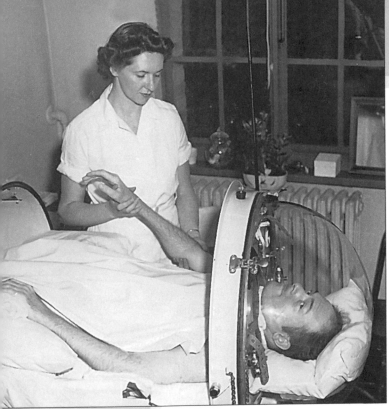

wondered if I could arrange for the same kind of service there that I had at the Baptist Hospital. I told her we could. She had a whole wing of a building that had not been used, and she said she would be willing to convert that into a polio ward if we could supply the equipment, the nurses, the doctors, and all of that. But we also needed to rewire the place. And we also needed to buy some refrigerators, to store the pharmaceuticals. So, I said, 'yes' to all of that without knowing. I knew we had to say 'yes'.

Were the doctors and nurses afraid to treat the polio patients?

I can't say that they were afraid to do it. But as soon as we imported the professionals from outside, this problem disappeared.

Where did the professionals come from?

Nurses and doctors were recruited by the American Red Cross, under a grant from the March of Dimes. The Joint Orthopedic Nursing Association and American Physical Therapy Association were involved with grants from the March of Dimes, doing the training of these people in the art of taking care of polio patients. We recruited nurses from all over the country, and we had to find a place for them to live, so we made the arrangements at one of the hotels in Little Rock to put them up. That lasted about one day before the hotel manager called us and said that the other guests in the hotel were concerned about contagion, and wondered if we couldn't do something about it. So we arranged for the nurses to change out of their uniforms at the hospital before they went to the hotel, so that they would not be recognized. We had been assured that they were not sources of contagion. There was a psychological problem that we were dealing with.

Talk about some of the March of Dimes efforts, such as the respiratory centers.

The respiratory centers naturally grew out of the initial respirator wards that were set up in hospitals because, unless something was done to get these patients weaned away from the respirators, you would simply be housing a lot of patients. You would finally run out of space, putting aside the humanitarian aspects. It would just be a logistical nightmare. The March of Dimes set up more than dozen respirator centers—Houston, Los Angeles, Minnesota, Ann Arbor, New York, all over the place. They were multidisciplinary centers where the whole focus was to get these people free of the dependency of the respirator. You had the physical therapists, the orthopedists, pediatricians, and all the people on the team working together with the one thing in mind: We have to restore this person to some kind of ability to survive outside the respirator. But there was the question of what to do for the long-term cases. There were more than a thousand cases that just could not be weaned away from the respirator. So the March of Dimes then started investing in respirator technology that allowed some of the patients to be taken care of at home. One of the innovations was a chest respirator, which was a big plastic shell that fit around the chest with this hose that went in, almost like a portable vacuum cleaner that would enable the patient to walk around the house instead of being trapped in this lung, looking at the ceiling all day. Then there was the whole idea of home care that we hear a lot about today. In those days it was unheard of. The March of Dimes arranged to send the respirator and the patient home with the idea that they would be visited by trained technicians, who would keep the respirator going and

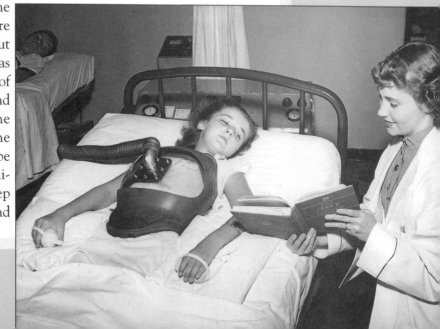

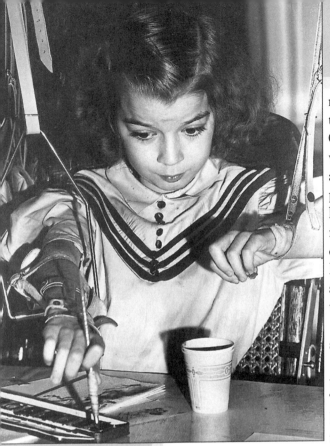

replace it if it was to wear out. So out of this center that I mentioned in Augusta, Georgia, they serviced the whole nation with home equipment of one kind or another. And this enabled a whole lot of people to survive at home who would not have otherwise been able to. There were no government programs that would handle this. There was no Medicaid, no Medicare. This was a service not unlike the services now available to kidney patients with dialysis.

What other services, outside respirator services, did the March of Dimes provide?

There were rehabilitation centers, where people could get long-term care. The biggest problem that the March of Dimes had, as these cases continued to mount and the number of survivors grew, was the fact that we weren't able to raise enough money just to give a blank check to everybody in the country, as we always had. With hospitals, it had always been that if you had polio, they accepted you, and they sent the bill to the March of Dimes. This began to be a real financial burden as time went on. So there was a conscious effort to look at each one of these families to see which ones needed to benefit from those services.

We also set up a regional system of social workers who would make visits to the homes that had a polio patient, and deal with all kinds of family issues. A whole lot of people felt guilt. Families felt that something they had done or hadn't done had caused this person, their child, to get polio. So there was a whole lot of trauma involved and we had social workers going to deal with that.

Let's talk about the porchlight campaign.

The public was willing to do almost anything to get rid of the problem of polio. The porchlight campaign was designed to have people

turn on their porchlights to signal that they wanted a campaign solic-
itor to come to the door. This was a case in which the people who
lived there invited the solicitors to come in and many times they
would invite them in the house to have coffee. That was the kind of
spirit that prevailed at that time, and it was reflective of how fundraising was. In those days you could just put a coin container in a store and
it would fill up in a week's time. Or in the early days there were actually little cards you could send out for one-cent postage, and people
could put dimes in the slots and send those back. Imagine how impossible that would be today.

What other methods did you have to raise funds?

Everyone went to the movies in those days, and Hollywood had a
very close connection with the March of Dimes, so through that connection they would actually stop the movies, turn on the lights, and
have people pass canisters up and
down the aisle, just like they
were going to church. And
nobody complained about stopping a movie right in the middle
and turning the lights on and
having a pitch for the fight
against polio. You didn't have the
resistance to fundraising, you
didn't have to make a sales pitch,
you didn't have to really convince them that this was a good
cause. They were already sensi-
tized to that. The campaign was
built all around Franklin Roosevelt's birthday in January. We
could start the campaign on the
first day of January, and pretty
much at the end of January, it
was over and of course now you
have to raise money year round.

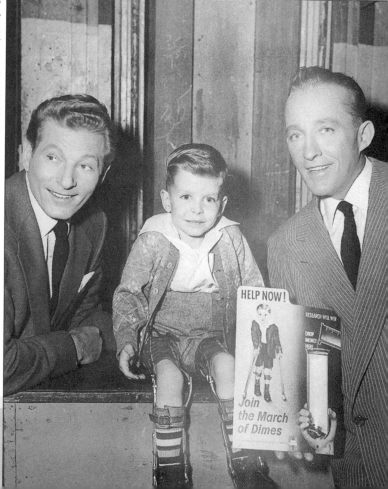

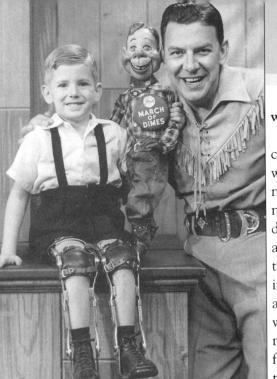

Tell me about the poster children and what that was all about.

Every parent of every poster child wanted that child to be associated with the March of Dimes. It was almost like a beauty contest in every community. Which child would be selected would depend not just on their appearance, but on the ability to deal with the public, to represent and to be an ambassador for the March of Dimes. We found that the parents were actually promoting their children in this contest, and we were very concerned not to appear like we were exploiting these children. So we would go through all kinds of maneuvers. We would meet with the parents, we'd meet with friends of the family, and so forth, to be sure that this was something they wanted to do.

How did you deal with the delicate relationship between the need to raise money and the hope that something would come from the money, i.e., a vaccine?

The epidemic occurred in Arkansas in 1949, and that same year Jonas Salk was opening up his laboratory in Pittsburgh. He now knew that a vaccine was possible and this word was very carefully protected because nobody wanted to send a premature announcement. It was a careful campaign to give our volunteers the suggestion that we're making progress, so as to give them some sense that their efforts were not in vain, but that we didn't know how long it will take. But to be honest, most of the people were supporting the March of Dimes because of its response to the epidemics. We had a national equipment pool in Augusta, Georgia, so equipment would be sent to wherever an epidemic struck, so that each community didn't have to maintain, on a standby basis, enough equipment to take care of an epidemic. Things like that were in the newspapers, constantly reminding everybody that the March of Dimes was providing all of these services for all of these patients, and I think that was almost enough to carry the campaign. But then as the vaccine began to be more and more likely, we began to plant the seeds with the volunteers that, 'Yeah, we're making progress,' and this gave a necessary lift. We later had to raise extra money for the vaccine's field trials in 1954. The March of Dimes made a calculated risk, spending $9 million with pharmaceutical companies on a vaccine that hadn't yet been licensed. So hypothetically it could have been $9 million down the drain, so it was kind of exciting times. The volunteers were aware we were investing in the production of this vaccine even though it hadn't been approved yet. Almost everybody in the March of Dimes family—the volunteers, the staff—had a feeling of expectancy, and that feeling was transformed into even more financial support.

Who were the volunteers?

The volunteers were really the homemakers. They came from almost everywhere because everybody felt an excitement about the prospect of doing something for this terrible problem. The patriotism of World War II still carried over into civilian activities, but this particular cause brought more women into the picture. The March of Dimes had affil-

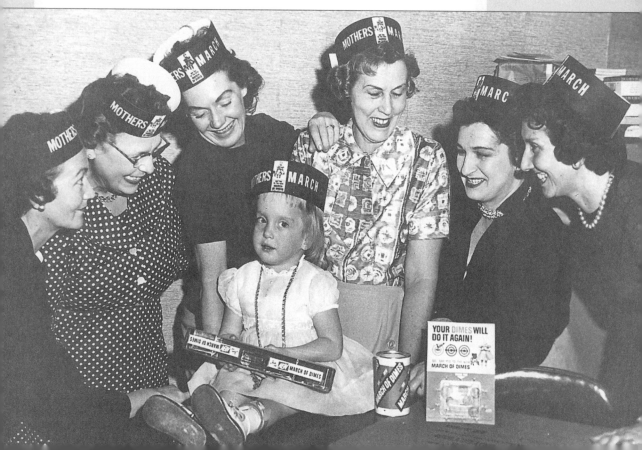

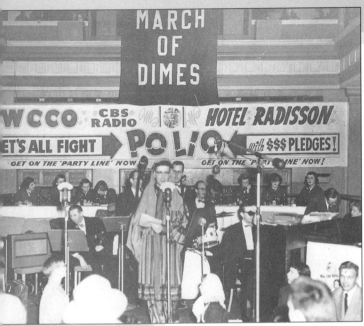

iations with PTAs, with business and professional women, with all kinds of library clubs, and with all kinds of organizations of women. Most of the men were already tied to the Rotary Club or Kiwanis Club or the Junior Chamber of Commerce, all kinds of organizations of men that had been involved in the war effort so they were already conditioned to do civic work. This brought the mothers into the picture. So you had whole families that were committed, and that was the way things were done in the 1950s.

Why was it the women who got involved?

Well, because the women in those days weren't in the work place the way they are today. They were at home and they had some time on their hands. Also, you're dealing with the lives of children, you're dealing with the same little Johnny they sent to school every day.

Tell me about the Cutter incident.

The Cutter incident was a dramatic setback in the field trials. Because everyone going into the field trials had been assured of the safety of the vaccine, the only thing in question was the efficacy. And so when the Cutter incident occurred and the publicity from Walter Winchell and other people ensued, it was a very shocking time for all of us at the March of Dimes. We were assured by all of the scientific people that this was some kind of aberration. But nobody knew what kind it was. Dr. Salk's first response was, 'Well, it has to be in the manufacturing process.' That was his immediate response, and that turned out to be the case. The Cutter laboratories, for whatever reason, somehow did not follow the protocols of Dr. Salk correctly, and some of the vaccine that they produced turned out to have some live virus in it. And some of the cases were actually caused by this. This, of course, was not only shocking to all of us, but it was very dramatic proof on the part of some of the naysayers that we never should have done this in the first place; we never should have undertaken this dramatic field study. We should have waited until things had been perfected and maybe another type of vaccine had been produced. So all the people who raised questions about the killed-virus vaccine in the first instance were beating the drums that this proved that they were right. So we had to identify that this was, in fact, a manufacturing error. Cutter had to admit that. And Cutter then had to deal with all the legal implications of that. But it enabled the field studies to continue to the point of conclusion.

Did it make people afraid of the vaccine?

The Cutter incident may have caused some people to be concerned about the vaccine. My own observation, and I think this was shared by most of my colleagues, was that they were not afraid of the vaccine after it was announced. The reason that it wasn't immediately used as widely as you might think was because that people simply psychologically felt the polio problem was solved. They almost had a psychological immunity because of the existence of the vaccine. So we had the crazy job of convincing people that had been praying for a vaccine, 'Hey, use it.' We went through three years of promoting immunization campaigns, for example.

What about the development of the Sabin vaccine?

Dr. Sabin was a recipient of a March of Dimes grant at the same time Dr. Salk was a recipient. So in a sense, even though neither one would like it characterized this way, it was kind of a race between the two of them. With the March of Dimes supporting both of the horses. Dr. Salk was the first horse that produced the vaccine, so March of Dimes decided we've got to use this one. But the March of Dimes support also continued for Dr. Sabin even beyond that. The only thing that the March of Dimes objected to was Dr. Sabin's idea that maybe his vaccine should

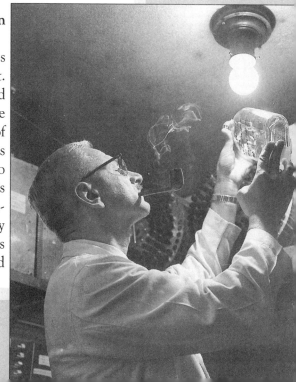

now be used on top of the Salk vaccine or after the Salk vaccine. And we took the position that this would, in a sense, taint the results. You never would have a separate outcome if you used both of them. So Dr. Sabin went to the Soviet Union and found a population there that was free of any taint. And he proved his vaccine effective by the same methods. By the time all this happened, though, about the late 1950s, the polio epidemics were a thing of the past. The numbers of cases in this country were relatively small and sporadic, and they did not amount to a public health problem.

What was the impact of the Salk vaccine on fundraising for the March of Dimes?

The first reaction was one of complete euphoria. The excitement was almost unbelievable. There was a feeling of pride in having accomplished something this miraculous. It was the first time it had ever been done by any volunteer agency. Now, following that, comes the problem of dealing with the distribution of the vaccine so that it is actually used effectively. But the March of Dimes fundraising results began to taper off, and we found that people thought the problem had been solved. There was no more fear of an epidemic. So the fear factor, as I call it, had disappeared from the fundraising. So what you're raising money for now was the reputation of the organization, the vaccine victory, but you have removed one of the primary motivations of fund raising, which was fear. So ironically, the success of the vaccine produced a negative effect on public support. We went through that process of trying to remind people that first of all, the job isn't over. We have thousands of polio cases still in hospitals that still need assistance. So, at the very peak of its popularity, the organization was facing a form of bankruptcy because its financial commitments were so great. We had $7 million in unpaid polio debts, and yet the public support began to drop off. Nobody in the public knew about that, but for people like me, who were working for the March of Dimes, it was a serious problem.

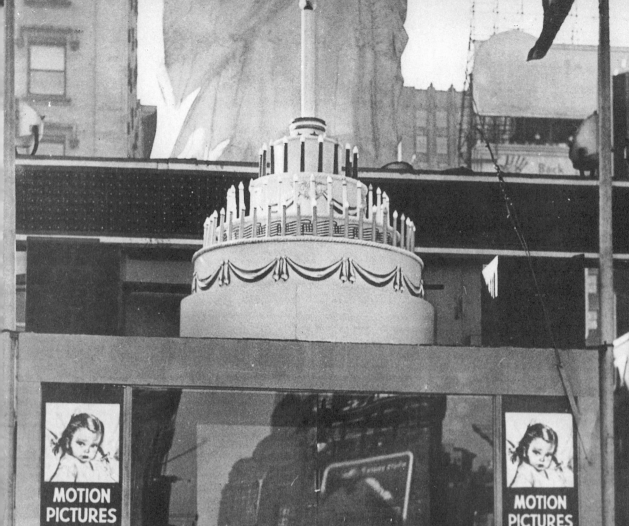

MOTION
PICTURES
1945
MARCH
of
DIMES

MOTION
PICTURES
1945
MARCH
of
DIMES

MARCH OF DIMES

MOTION PICTURES WAR ACTIVITIES COMMITTEE *New York Area*

Give IN THE NAME
OF YOUR CHILD

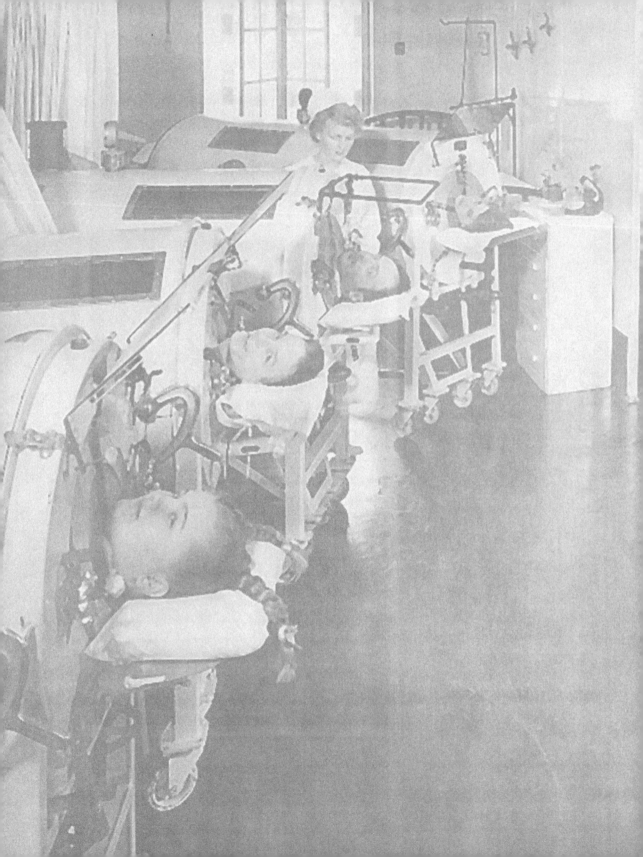

Chapter 4

The Polio Patient

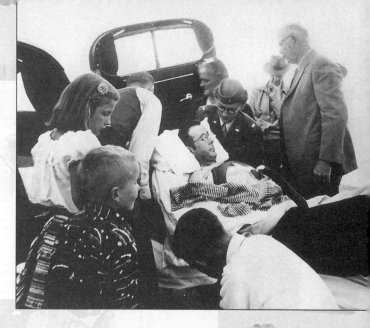

I could hear my mother on the telephone, calling the doctor hour after hour and she kept getting delays. And she just kept calling. And then she came back and she'd try to assure me that I was going to be all right. I remember crying a lot because I was so frightened. What is wrong with me? Was I dying? Is this something really bad, Mom? I didn't say the word either. I didn't say polio. It was a horrendous fear. I was just afraid I was going to die. Then that evening my mother went to the phone again, and I could hear the fear in her voice. And she ordered the doctor: 'You come here, and you come here right now because I don't know what to do for her.' And then he came . . . and then I heard him say to my mother and dad, 'I'm afraid Charlene has infantile paralysis.' I remember crying, just crying. I was convinced I was going to die, this was a death sentence. My mother started crying, I heard her crying. My father said, 'Are you saying she has polio? And the doctor said, 'Yes.' And my dad said, 'Are you sure?' And he said, 'Yes', and he went on to say, 'We've got to get her to a polio hospital tonight.'

—Charlene Pugleasa,
polio survivor

99

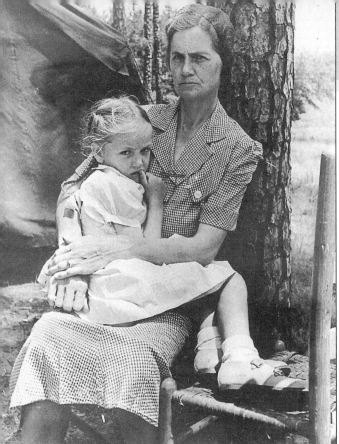

Most epidemic diseases pass through a region with the sudden fury of a violent storm. They cut a swath of devastation and vanish, leaving a legacy of mass graves and then mass amnesia. The influenza pandemic of 1918 killed over twenty-one million people, including 675,000 in the United States and thousands more American soldiers stationed abroad, but it was hardly remembered ten years later. Poliomyelitis was different, however. It's victims were far fewer, but most survived, and many required a lifetime of care.

Like every aspect of this newly recognized disease, the question of how to care for polio patients was a confusing mystery. Even diagnosis was difficult. The first symptoms were mild and deceptive. A chill, a slight fever, a general sense of fatigue, were all that many ever felt. The statistics on polio epidemics must be read with the knowledge that as many as 90 percent of those who were infected never even knew it, and so they were never recorded among the ill.

For the unlucky minority who were clearly sick, the disease progressed into an acute stage that was as terrifying as it was unpredictable. The early fever might abate—or it might give way to extreme pain, muscle weakness, and paralysis. The paralysis might or might not be temporary. Recovery might come within days, or weeks, or even months; tales of sudden improvements long after the onset of disease fed the hopes of many disabled patients for months and even years after they were injured.

The most lethal form of the disease, bulbar polio, caused paralysis of the muscles that regulate breathing, so that the body literally forgot how to perform this most vital and automatic of functions. In 1928, Philip Drinker, an engineer at the Harvard School of Public Health, developed what soon became known as the "iron lung." Patients were laid on a mattress that was then rolled into a metal box, with only their heads, bound in a tight rubber collar, sticking out. A powerful motor pumped air in and out of the box, artificially inflating and deflating the patient's lungs. For many polio patients, the respite provided by the iron lung allowed them to survive the most acute stage of polio inflammation, after which they were able to breathe unassisted. Some were only in the iron lung for days. Others remained inside the respirator for weeks, and some never could go for long without mechanical help. Sadly, even with the help of the respirator, many died.

Over the years, the technology of the iron lung improved. Motors were quieted, cases were streamlined, mirrors were mounted on angled hinges from the top of the machine so that the patients, immobilized on their backs, could read or see people behind them. From the 1930s, the whooshing noise of the iron lung became the background music for the polio experience— prison and salvation, and the image of all that people feared most about the disease.

With no clear knowledge of how polio was contracted or how the virus caused paralysis, doctors felt justified in trying almost anything to stop the ravages of the disease. Patients were injected with the smallpox vaccine, adrenaline, horse, sheep, goat, and monkey serum, streptococcic serum, their own spinal fluid, their own blood, their parents' blood, convalescent serum extracted from recovered polio

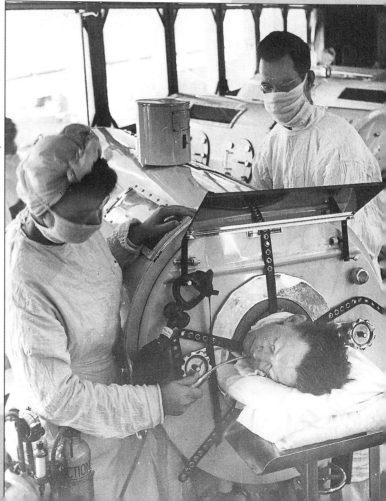

patients, and anything else their enterprising physicians thought might help. There were plasters, pills, and nasal sprays, some causing dire side effects, but none, alas, had any noticeable benefit. Some doctors thought that draining fluid from the spine might relieve pressure on the brain and spinal cord, thus reducing pain and paralysis. All these experimenters were elated to report good results, despite the painful nature of the procedure, but careful scientific analysis showed that the various treatments were never statistically better than doing nothing.

Yet another mystery of polio patient care was the question of how to control the physical distortion that was a frequent aftermath of the disease. As doctors studied the shortened legs, shriveled arms, or twisted spines that often followed an acute polio infection, they concluded that paralysis on one side of the body left muscles too weak to maintain normal alignment. Without the elaborate balance of the symmetrical muscular system, it was thought, the patient's body would be stretched and pulled out of shape like a loosely knit sweater carelessly flung over a fence to dry. To avoid this physical distortion, most doctors recommended immobilization during the period of acute infection. Arms, legs, and spine were held rigid with wooden splints, then were confined in plaster casts for weeks or even months at a time.

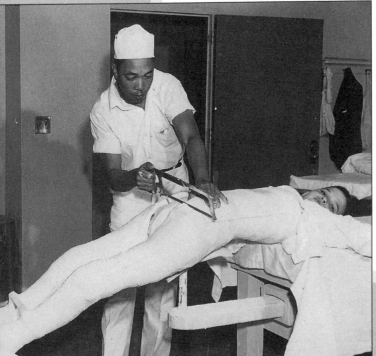

Rigid containment was accompanied by complete inactivity. Doctors warned patients, in the sternest terms, to avoid muscle manipulation or stimulation with electric currents. Months of bed rest were essential for any hope of recovery, they said. Massage was harmless after the acute stage was over, the experts concluded, but exercise would only further develop muscles on one side of the body, leading to more twisting and bodily distortion. Exercises like the warm-water workouts Roosevelt enjoyed at Warm Springs, or even the necessary training to walk with braces or crutches, were considered best when postponed for eighteen months to two years after recovery from the initial infection.

Given this regimen, many polio patients emerged from convalescence with atrophied limbs and diminished power in their non-paralyzed muscles. Until the 1940s, much of the treatment for polio patients consisted of retraining these remaining muscles so that paralytics could at least use the burgeoning array of arm, leg, and neck braces, crutches, and wheelchairs that had been devised to meet their needs.

The modern era of polio rehabilitation started in 1940, with the arrival in the United States of an eccentric Australian nursing sister named Elizabeth Kenny. Working independently of any medical center, Kenny had devised her own system of care for polio patients, a regimen of hot packs and massage that worked best when started in the very early stages of the disease. A large, forthright, authoritative woman, she insisted that all of the American experts were wrong and that the characteristic muscle twisting of the polio patient came from the spasm of affected muscles, not their stretching. Therefore, the proper treatment was to relieve the spasms as soon as they occurred, using heat and repetitive muscle manipulation.

Kenny's methods were not well received at first. Nobody knew anything about this strange, brusque woman from the other side of the world, and doctors were wary of quack cures and untried methods. Still, Kenny attracted enough support to establish a clinic at Minneapolis General Hospital, in Minnesota. Trials of the so-called Kenny Method showed such clear benefits that, in a few years, immobilization was all but abandoned. For the polio patients of the 1940s and 1950s, a new sensation was added to the aftermath of polio. The tormenting rigidity of plaster was replaced by the distinctive smell of steaming vats of woolen cloths, the primitive but effective hot packs, that eased the pain of twisted muscles.

As the toll of polio epidemics rose, it did so in all parts of American society. Black children were struck down as often as whites, but in the still racially segregated south, black polio victims were turned away from hospitals and from Warm Springs and were told to seek help elsewhere. For them the National Foundation funded the Infantile Paralysis Center at Tuskegee Institute in Alabama. The children there received the same treatment that was recommended by the National Foundation at all of the rehabilitation centers it supported, but many of the Tuskegee patients suffered from having to travel so far to receive necessary care. Many others never were able to make the trip. The era of polio epidemics ended before the era of desegregation began, and "separate but sometimes equal" was the best that could be said about polio patient care in America. The National Foundation was dedicated to helping polio patients, but not to changing the world.

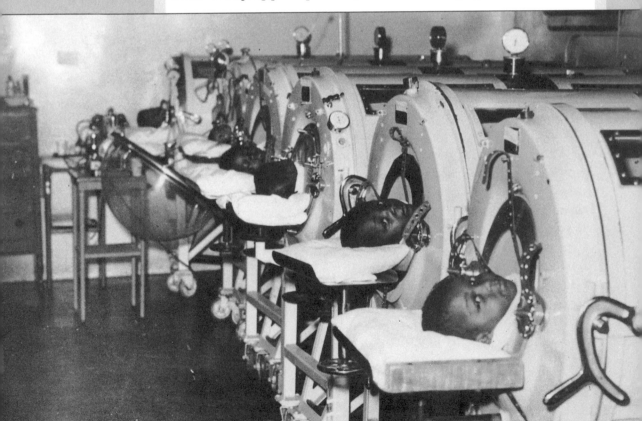

Voices
Mark O'Brien

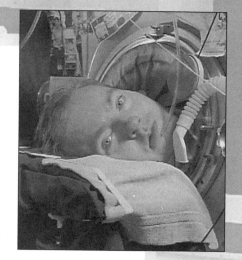

Mark O'Brien was six years old in 1955 when he came down with polio in Boston. He was in a coma for thirty days. He stayed in the hospital for two years. After a series of illnesses, he was put back into the lung at age eleven, where he has lived most of his life.

Go back to 1955, to the moment you knew something was wrong.

I was six years old in 1955 when I got polio. I was sleeping in the top of the bunk bed I shared with my brother Ken, and I had a pain in my belly. I waited it out. Finally, I got the ladder to go down and I told my parents. They called the family doctor and he came out. The doctor thought I should go to Children's Hospital in Boston and then my father drove me and everyone in the family to the hospital. He told me when he was a little boy he had his appendix out at the same hospital. We had to wait a lot and go to different rooms. They told me to roll over onto the bed, and that's the last thing I remember. I passed out. I was in a coma for thirty days after that.

What did you see when you first woke up?

I don't remember what I saw when I first came out of the coma. But I was in a big, dark room with several beds and my teddy bear was on one of the beds nearby. I must have been quite confused. I don't remember those early days. I told that to a psychology professor once. He said it's probably just as well. My parents visited me often, but a lot of times I'd see them entering the room and they'd disappear. I didn't know what was happening. Later, I heard that in the early stages of polio people have hallucinations, but no one told me and it was just so scary. I kept having audio hallucinations for like two years afterwards. I could hear my mother's voice when she wasn't really there.

You were part of an epidemic of polio in Massachusetts in 1955. Why didn't you get the vaccine?

I couldn't get the vaccine because there had been a bad batch of Salk vaccine released in Southern California. A lot of people got polio out of that. The governor of Massachusetts suspended the distribution of the Salk vaccine during September of 1955. And the rate of polio infection went way up, so near the end of the month the governor revoked that order. So I just had this little window of opportunity. That's why I got polio.

You were in the hospital for over two years. What do you remember about it?

There were a lot of children my age with polio. A lot of them were from out of state, a few from out of the country, and they seldom saw their parents. I saw my parents, my grandparents, aunts, and uncles a

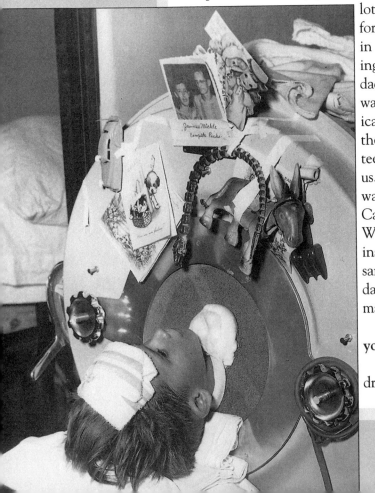

lot. The other children would scream for their parents all the time, especially in the evenings. They were either crying or yelling for their mommies and daddies. It was very hellish and scary. It was hard to keep it together. The physical therapists tried to be as kind as they could. There were hospital volunteers [who] read to us and played with us. They were a great comfort. There was a boy my age named Johnny Casper and he had the bed next to me. We talked together and sang and insulted the nurses. Every Friday we sang, 'Friday's fish day, we hate fish day, throw all the fish in the fisherman's face!'

Did your brothers and sisters visit you in the hospital?

I think they had a rule against children visiting, but I remember once, it might have been around Christmas of 1956, they put me on a gurney and took me down to the lobby. I saw Ken and Karen, my brother and sister, for the first time in a little over a year.

Where did you go from the hospital?

The convalescent hospital was owned by the big hospital. I was in a little room with two girls about the same age as I was. The three of us were in iron lungs. A huge difference [from the hospital] was that there was a big porch and we could go outside in the good weather. Most of the patients were teenagers. The teenagers were in rocking beds. They were less disabled than us little kids. They would have rock-and-roll going on WBZ Radio 103. And I remember the physical therapist, Nancy Warren, taught me about baseball that summer. Don Larson had pitched his no-hitter the year before and I was curious and she taught me all about it. I listened to the Red Sox games out on the porch.

You were very young. When did you realize what was happening to you?

At first I thought I'd get better. I mean, I knew I couldn't move my arms or legs, and I got real tired very fast. I was scared of being moved. I just thought I'd get better. My only experience with disease was getting colds or bumping around. My mother always used to kiss my knee when I skinned it. The nurses said that when I ate my broccoli, I'd get better. Or my asparagus or carrots. I believed it for a while. I don't remember when I stopped believing in it. I think it took me a couple of years to realize this was for life and it was very, very depressing to realize that. I saw other kids getting better around me. I once saw a kid who'd been in bed all the time learning how to walk without crutches and he was going right by me. I wasn't going anywhere. It was terrible to realize.

Tell me about going home, knowing this was permanent.

My parents had an option. My father checked out this highly recommended nursing home and found out that the life expectancy was like eighteen months. So they brought me home. I remember the day I came home. Ken and Karen had made all these signs saying, 'Welcome Home,' and my parents were very happy to see me. My father had installed an intercom to connect my room with my parents' room, which was the bedroom above me in the two-story house. I was very happy to get home. My mother would get me up every morning and put me on the ambulance cart and take me into the TV room. We'd watch cartoons, *Laurel and Hardy*, before Ken went to school. Then she'd put me back in my bed, wash me and everything, and watch TV and read. My father bought me a little portable, I guess in 1959 or 1960, except I always went to the TV room 'cause my father had this big twenty-four-inch set. I wanted to watch the Red Sox with him, so we watched the Red Sox every weekend.

Did you have friends?

I hung out with my brother's friends. There were a bunch of boys my age in the neighborhood and I watched them play baseball or football or kickball. There was a big vacant lot where we lived. My father would push me on the cart to the lot and I'd sit maybe twenty, thirty feet away from where the guys would stand. Sometimes they just had a pitcher, first baseman, and a left fielder, and sometimes my father and the father of one of my neighbors would play with us. But the boys were very curious and friendly. They treated me well.

Tell me about birthdays.

I really don't remember them well. Once, we'd set up a big birthday party with cake and ice cream out in the kitchen and I got sick. I just had to go back into the iron lung. I felt really bad about that. And I remember when I first got polio, they had a big Christmas tree set up in the courtyard of Children's Hospital. And for some reason they picked me to turn on the lights. I had to go out there at night, there were people from the TV channels. I think the mayor was there. I didn't know what was going on and I pushed a button and lit up the Christmas tree. It was very late at night, I remember I was sleepy.

I remember after we moved to California, my sister Rachel would bring the presents to me in my bedroom. They'd all be books. She was like six years old, she'd unwrap them and say 'Ooh, it's *Plato's Republic*! Oh boy!' She'd jump up and down. '*Plato's Republic*, oh boy!' Then she'd help take me into the living room where the tree was.

Were you in the iron lung all the time?

When I was in the hospital, they got me so I could stay out of the iron lung all day and then eventually all night too. I just used a chest respirator at night and I was able to go home a little with my parents. [But] I got sick, like every two months. I was throwing up, having diarrhea. My parents would have to take me back to Children's Hospital, they had to stick an IV in me. This went on for two or three years. Eventually the doctor said I should be back in the iron lung, and so they delivered an iron lung to our house. It just barely fit in my room.

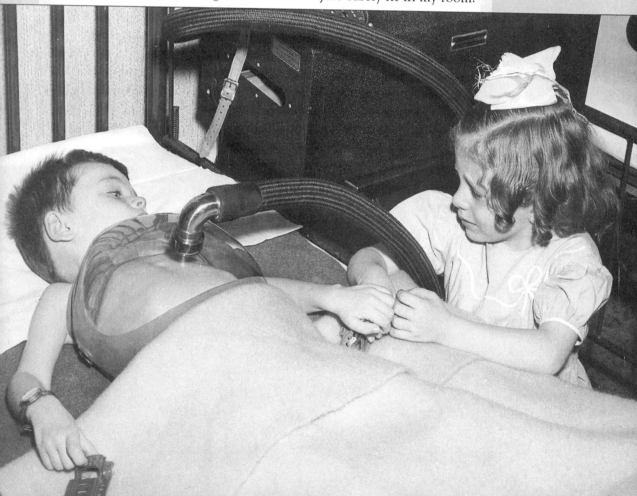

It was in 1960 or 1961, when I was eleven, when I went back in the iron lung. For a long time, until, oh, 1983, I just needed it at night. I could be out all day.

What about school?

The first few years when I was in the hospital, they had teachers working in the hospitals. After I came home, the town we lived in employed a teacher who visited children who were temporarily or permanently disabled. She'd come two or three days a week until I got to eighth grade, and then the junior high teachers would come after school and tutor me. When I came to California we did the same thing for the year. I think I got a pretty good education because I was working one-on-one with the teachers, and I was very eager to please them. I took a general equivalency diploma and passed that. And then, a million years after that I came to Berkeley. I graduated with a BA in English in 1983. I went to the graduate school of journalism for a year before the post-polio hit me and I had to drop out.

Tell me about your writing.

I think I wanted to be a writer since I was twelve or so. I saw an episode of *Leave It to Beaver* in which the Beaver decided he wanted to be a writer and I thought maybe I could do that. I know I was afraid of growing up 'cause I didn't know what grown-up people with polio did exactly. I didn't have any role models. When I was in the hospital in the 1970s, I was able to use a typewriter with fancy microswitches. My last quarter, when I was an undergraduate, I tried to get into a poetry writing class. I didn't think I'd be good enough, but I submitted my poems to the professor. He guided me, he encouraged me. I didn't think I could write but Peter L. Scott, the professor, gave me a lot of encouragement. Eventually the poems were collected and a book was published in 1990. *Breathing* is the name of the book. And that sold well, so I keep writing poems. I met a poet named Ronald McGowen, who once said, 'You should write more poetry about your life.' And he thumped the iron lung with his hand. He said, 'What's it like to be in here?' So I've been writing poems about disability. But I write about politics or people I've known, or family. I guess I write about whatever anyone else would write about.

About love?

Oh, yeah. Well, I write about whoever I happen to be in love with at the time. I've written very long love poems, very short love poems, and they're almost as hard to write as political poems. A few years ago I tried writing sonnets.

Do you write about loneliness?

Yeah, I suppose I did. 'The Man in the Iron Lung' is about loneliness in a way. I really don't think I write about loneliness in itself, it's more like missing people or being different from people.

Not about anger?

Oh, yeah, I have a few angry poems. I showed some of my poems to my brother once. He said, 'Are they all downers?' I said, 'Well, yes, most of them are downers.' I have a happy poem about a woman I was in love with once, the times we went out together. I wrote a poem about Jesus rowing across a lake, trying to get away from everyone, seeking isolation.

"The Man in the Iron Lung"
by Mark O'Brien

I scream
The body electric,
This yellow, metal, pulsing cylinder
Whooshing all day, all night
In its repetitious, dull mechanical rhythm.
Rudely it inserts itself in the map of my body,
which my midnight mind,
Dream drenched cartographer of terra incognita,
Draws upon the dark parchment of sleep.
I scream
In my body electric;
A dream snake bites my left leg.
Indignant I shake the gods by their abrupt shoulders,
    Demanding to know how such a vile slitherer
Could enter my serene metal shell.
The snake is punished with death,
The specialty of the gods.
Clamped up still in my leg,
It must be removed;
The dream of the snake
Must be removed,
While I am restored
By Consciousness, that cruelest of gods.
In metal hard reluctance
To my limited, awkward, declasse
Body electric
As it whispers promises of health,
Whooshes beautiful lies of invulnerability.
Size, similarly, seraphically, relentlessly.
It is me,
It is me.

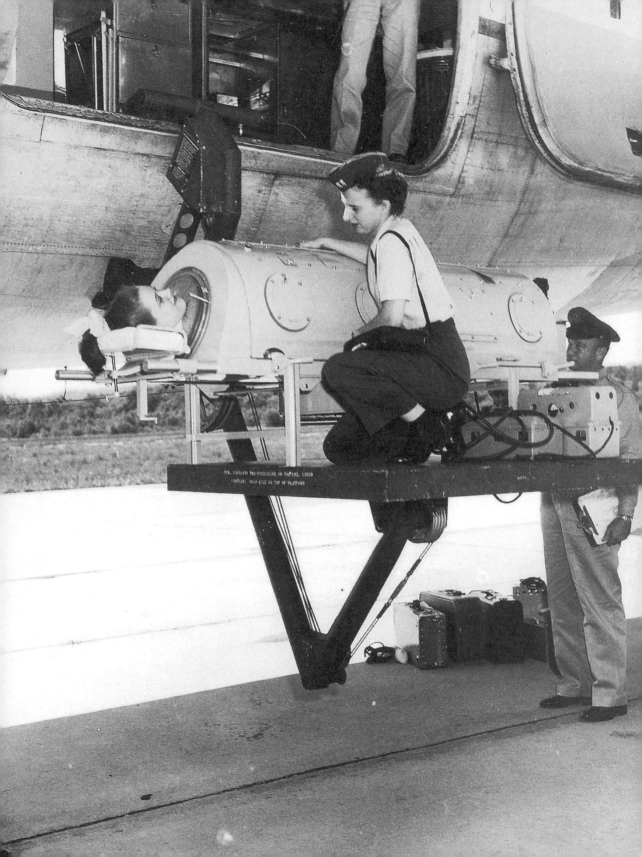

Richard Aldrich, M.D.

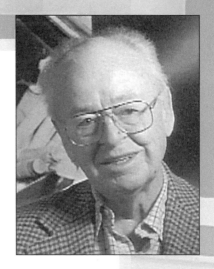

Dr. Richard Aldrich was a resident at the University of Minnesota Hospital during the epidemics of 1948 and 1949. He had just come back from World War II and likened the epidemic summers in the hospitals to his experience in combat.

What are your memories of the epidemic in Minnesota?

The first summer when I was home in Minnesota [after serving in World War II] was that gosh-awful polio epidemic they had there. We admitted 464 proven cases of polio just at the University Hospital, which is unbelievable. And this was a very severe paralytic form. Maybe two or three hours after a lot of these kids would come in with a stiff neck or a fever, they'd be dead. It was unbelievable. It was just loads of people that came in, sometimes with only a fever but usually a headache and a little stiffness in the neck. And just absolutely terrified. At the height of the epidemic, the people in Minneapolis were so frightened that there was nobody in the restaurants. There was practically no traffic, the stores were empty. It just was considered a feat of bravado almost to go out and mingle in public. A lot of people just took up and moved away, went to another city. It was really a disaster.

How did the hospital handle so many patients?

They cleared whole wards. I remember there was a room 43, and another one, 33. They had nothing but polio there. The hospital just made it happen. I've never seen anything like it in the rest of my life. But can you admit 464 kids into one hospital? So we had to get the other hospitals in town involved in this. And then we took some of our people who had learned a lot about polio, and they began to run the polio unit in the other hospitals. Another feature that was important was that they had somebody named Drinker who had invented the Philip Drinker respirator. And there weren't enough of them, so they had to bring them in by air from all over the country. The people were flying in extra respirators. So we had big rooms in the hospital with maybe ten of these respirators going. And you had to have somebody sitting there monitoring them, so that if the electricity went off a patient wouldn't die. We got very, very good at it over a period of a few weeks.

We organized our service at the University Hospital so that we had someone there in person twenty-four hours a day. We had a steady stream of patients coming in, and they were mostly children, but there were some adults. And we divided up into two teams, with a nurse and another attendant, and we'd take a history in three or four minutes. You could tell what the story was. And then we'd do a spinal tap, which we got to be awfully good at, we were doing so many. And then we had another team that, as soon as the spinal fluid would drip

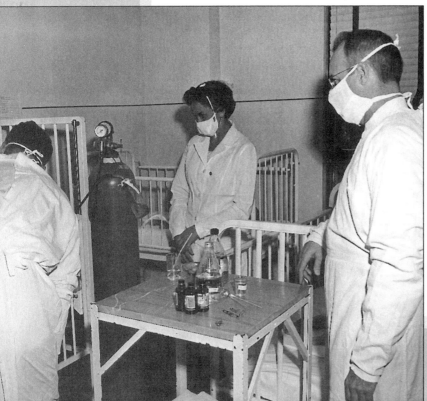

in these little test tubes, they would take it just around the corner where they had a nice laboratory all set up. And they'd do the cell counts and call us and we'd know right away whether the cells were there for a polio diagnosis. Then you had to assess what kind of paralysis the person had, or if they didn't have any, what to expect.

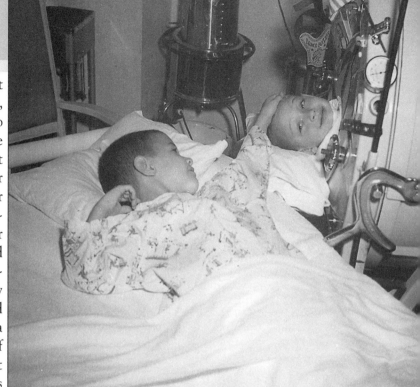

And then the worst part of the whole thing came, and that's when you had to talk to the parents. Those were some of the most awful experiences I ever had in my life; I've never forgotten them. It was sitting down with a mother and a father whose child you just diagnosed as having polio. They didn't know what to expect. [You had to] reassure them that a very high percentage of these kids were going to get well, which the statistics showed, and the chances of death were small, too. And you had to be convincing, you couldn't bluff anybody. But you had to tell them there was an extra risk if there were signs of involvement with the cranial nerves, what's called bulbar polio. That was really very serious.

When you were telling one kid's folks, more kids were being wheeled through the door. How did the doctors and nurses deal with it?

We organized ourselves so that what we called the first team was there all the time. We had to spell each other so that we could go to sleep for four to six hours. It was like being in combat. You have to be on the ball and ready to go all the time. You were tired, exhausted, and frightened at the same time. We didn't want to get polio ourselves. We were all concerned as heck about it because we'd bring it home. Two of my kids had polio, fortunately with no paralysis, but I'm sure I brought it home to them. You couldn't avoid it. Because you were covered with saliva, you'd bring it with you.

For those of us who had to deal with the epidemic, we had very little time off, we didn't have any schedule anymore. We just decided that we would work until we were just absolutely bone tired. And we'd get somebody to relieve us and go and get four hours of sleep and something to eat. Nobody had any hours off; it was just taboo. In fact, your colleagues would just be really angry. You were essentially on call all the time. It was a total emergency day and night, day after day after day for weeks, and we all lost a lot of weight. Some of the residents and the interns I was with were almost cracked up over it. I remember in particular one very sensitive lady. She just dissolved in tears for a day or two because it was so awful. A lot of people were so overwhelmed by the polio epidemic that they literally couldn't function. They'd just curl up in bed and stay there. It was that bad.

The combat image is poignant since this was just after the end of World War II. Was that a factor?

We had about twenty-five interns and residents on our service. And out of that group I'd say about six or eight were women, the rest were men. And nearly all the men had been in some kind of combat in the Air Force or the Army or the Navy, and I don't know if I should use the word hardened, but they knew what it was like to have to suffer. And that was a very important ingredient. And they also were, I think, much more sensitive to the needs of patients and the parents than they would've been otherwise. The experience of the war had changed how they felt about their fellow man quite a bit. I know it did me, and I think almost all the rest of them were influenced the same way. So that you had a big team with experience, with specialized skills, that really knew what we were doing.

What were those special skills or techniques?

One of the first things we discovered, which was brand new, was that with kids that develop bulbar polio, early intervention with pressured oxygen was essential. There was a guy from the Mayo clinic named Elmholtz who was an expert. He'd done a lot of work for the Air Force on pressure oxygen masks and he came up and joined us. The Elmholz contribution was to put a tracheotomy tube into these kids early on, and nobody ever did this before. And then you could give pressure oxygen, raise the oxygen level in their circulation, which turned out to be extremely important in blocking the degree of paralysis. Apparently, your nerve cells are very sensitive to lack of oxygen. And we learned this clinically just by the observations we made. All of a sudden we were very sure that we were saving a lot of kids that would otherwise have died because of the pressure-oxygen thing. And saving people from very severe damage that would really make their lives miserable. And that was a dramatic change. Everything was jury-rigged—we weren't sure what to do next—but that really did work.

Some of us were discovering things that were brand new. Nobody had faced this before, where you would see as many cases of this and you're with

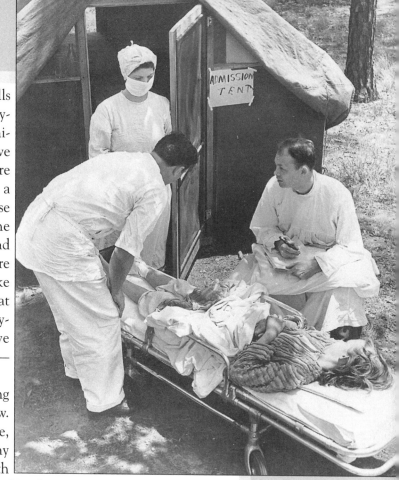

them day and night for weeks. You begin to see subtle changes. We found, for example, although it sounds peculiar, that kids who were going to get bulbar polio, who were really in danger, would get this red flush to their eyes. There are other symptoms that nobody ever connected. One of the most common characteristics was that their voice quality would change. Something was being done to their vocal cords. You'd listen for these very, very subtle things, and boy, when this happened and you put the pressure oxygen on, you really threw the book at them. Because if you could get those bulbar symptoms early, you could save the kid from very serious damage.

How did the epidemic progress?

As the summer went on, the severity of the bulbar cases got worse and worse and worse and worse and we kept saying, 'My God, I hope we get a frost.' We were completely beat, when suddenly the first frost came in the fall, and with that the epidemic dropped off in no time flat. We had new cases coming in, and we had all the old cases to deal with, but not this influx.

Sister Kenny was a significant figure in Minnesota during the epidemics. Tell me about her.

Sister Kenny was a delight. She arrived with a little bit of advance publicity. She's a big lady, probably weighs about 190 pounds, strong, big arms, not chubby, but just big and strong, you know, like a good blocking back at Notre Dame. Sister Kenny, she really knew her stuff. She taught us how to use the hot packs properly, and we began to use the Kenny hot-pack treatment, along with a lot of other things we did. It was dramatic to me. I had a question about whether it worked or not. But once I saw how well it worked, I had no problem with it. It made the kids much more comfortable. And she circulated around, supervising, seeing that the hot-pack stuff was done properly. She was a real asset to the whole show. And her personality was a big asset, too, because she was a tough cookie. She wouldn't take anything from anybody. She was just a real, hard-boiled person because she knew her stuff and you couldn't get her to modify it, which was probably a good thing.

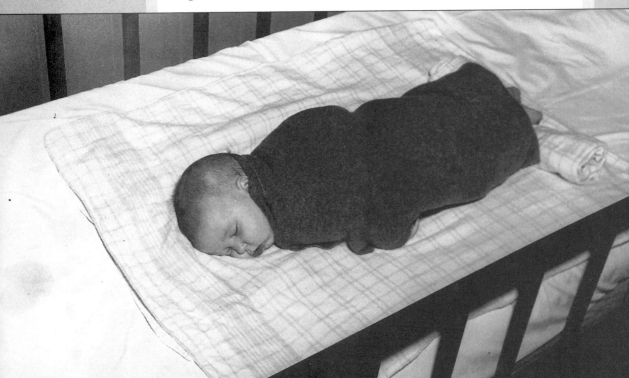

Charlene Pugleasa

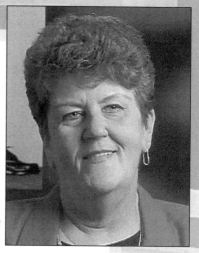

Charlene Pugleasa was thirteen years old when she contracted polio while living in Virginia, Minnesota.

Can you tell me about your first symptoms of polio?

It was September of 1953, and I had just turned thirteen. I'd had a big slumber party a week before, which was really kind of a scary thing to have because it was polio season. But it was the end of polio season so parents were more relaxed and more willing to let girls get together. I mention that because there were so many of us at this party, and a week later I started feeling sick. Friday night is when I knew I was getting sick, but I thought this was something very minor. On Saturday our family went to do school shopping, and my two cousins, my brother, and I were all in the back seat. My brother was twelve and he was poking at me and I remember screaming, getting very upset. Just to touch me my skin hurt really bad, so when he poked me in the ribs, or touched me anywhere, it was just awful. I think he thought I was just joking.

We lived in Sudan, Minnesota, and once a week, we girls walked two miles to the one and only theater. And I talked my mother into letting me go. *Above and Beyond* was the name of the movie, with Robert Taylor. I don't remember much about the movie. I only remember being real sick in the movie. My back ached, my body hurt, and it became more than just annoying, it was a piercing pain, a bad headache, sore throat. Walking home it was another two-mile walk. And when we walked home, my girlfriends had to keep slowing down and they kept asking me what was the matter. Nothing felt paralyzed, nothing. You know, I didn't think polio. I was just tired; my legs just didn't want to carry me. I got home that night and I got sicker on Saturday night.

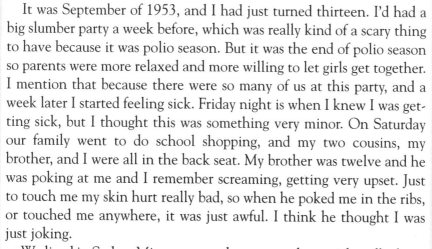

Sunday and Monday were probably the longest days of my life. My mother had been in contact with the local doctor, calling, calling, calling, 'What's the matter with our daughter?' The doctor had seen me, and didn't know what was wrong. I'm of Finnish heritage, and Finnish people believe in Finnish saunas. And my parents had an island on Lake Vermilion and there was a sauna on that island. My mother and dad decided to bundle me up, and the whole family went off to the island. The wood stove was heated in the sauna, and I took a sauna with my cousin. It was so hot she was driven right out. And I was so cold I was shaking. I was having a hard time moving. My mother came down to the sauna and got me dressed. And then she and my father wrapped blankets around me and they helped me up to the cabin. All of the woolen quilts my mother had made were hauled out and they were piled up on me. And I was still shaking. I remember the bed shaking, I remember crying, I remember being scared and asking, 'What's the matter with me? What's the matter with me?' I'm told that I sort of went in and out of consciousness because my fever was so high. My mother tried to get hot broth down me and I couldn't. I would vomit it. We got back that night, and I couldn't get upstairs, my legs were too weak to carry me up the stairs. My back was in too much pain. The muscles were pulling backward. No one could touch me because I hurt so bad.

My parents called the doctor that evening, and got me bundled up and to the hospital. We had the little local hospital with one doctor. And I saw the doctor that night and he didn't know what was wrong with me. He thought I possibly had a kidney infection, so he took a

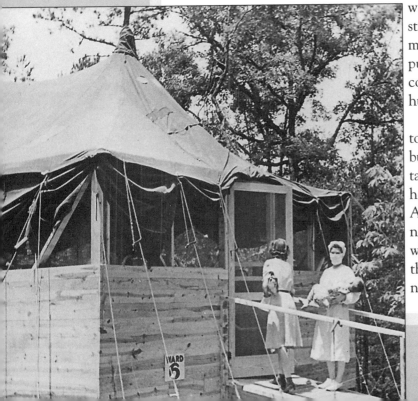

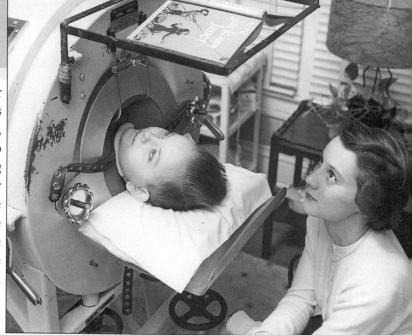

urine sample. I remember thinking maybe this was something really dreaded, because I had never been so sick. I believe from talking to my mother years later that she feared from the onset that this was what we were dealing with, but she didn't mention it. But the doctor thought the word polio wasn't even used anymore. I was thirteen and he was concerned because I hadn't had my period yet. And I remember thinking that I didn't like this business at all. You know, if this is what becoming a woman is all about I don't want it. He told my mother to put cold compresses on my forehead. I know my fever had gotten up to 104, and there was also nausea. So I got back on this studio hide-a-bed and I was no longer writhing in pain because I felt I was too weak. And what was happening was that my body would just twist and pull backwards. She put these cold compresses on me to try and get the fever down, and even that hurt. Now she wanted to massage my muscles but it was too awful.

On Monday morning, my brother and cousins went to school. My father was starting his midnight shift and he usually went to bed early in the morning, and he didn't. I could tell he was worried. I could hear my mother on the telephone, calling the doctor hour after hour and she kept getting delays. And she just kept calling. And then she came back and she'd try to assure me that I was going to be all right. I remember crying a lot because I was so frightened. What is wrong with me? Was I dying? Is this something really bad, Mom? I didn't say the word either. I didn't say polio. It was a horrendous fear. I was just afraid I was going to die.

Then that evening my mother went to the phone again, and I could hear the fear in her voice. And she ordered the doctor: 'You come here, and you come here right now because I don't know what to do for her.' And then he came. When he came in he stood there, and he looked at me, he just stood there with his hand on his chin. And then he told my mother that I didn't have a kidney infection. I was puzzling him. So he asked me to lift my head up, and I couldn't and then he put his hands back here to lift my head up. And I screamed, I just screamed in pain because the muscles in the back of my neck were so bad. And that's all he did. Then he uncovered me and he lifted one leg at a time. And when he raised my leg I screamed. I remember that pain shooting right up through my leg and up my back, and up my neck and up into my head.

And then he said to my mother, 'Just cover her up and get Charlie. I want to talk to you.' My mother ran upstairs and got my dad and they came down, and then I heard him say to my mother and dad, 'I'm afraid Charlene has infantile paralysis.' I remember crying, just crying. I was convinced I was going to die, this was a death sentence. My mother started crying, I heard her crying. My father said, 'Are you saying she has polio?' And the doctor said, 'Yes.' And my dad said, 'Are you sure?' And he said, 'Yes,' and he went on to say, 'We've got to get her to a polio hospital tonight.'

The town had one ambulance and it was on a call. [The doctor] told my parents that they had to drive me because we couldn't wait for it to come back. I remember being all covered up in blankets and them trying to get me in the back seat to lie down, and I couldn't because I was in too much pain. And I couldn't sit up because my muscles wouldn't hold me up. And I remember the doctor saying, 'If you sit her right between the two of you it will hold her up.' And that's what they did. And I sat so straight, and my head was pulled so back. That was about a sixty-mile ride and I felt every bump, every railroad track. And my mother and father and I cried and talked about polio. My mother kept saying, 'Well, maybe it's not. The doctor said you have to have your spine tapped. Maybe it's not polio.'

Tell me about that moment when you learned you had polio.

When I heard my father say 'polio,' what went through my mind was all those miles of film footage that I remember seeing. We went to the theater often, we didn't have television. And before the movie there was always the newsreel, which carried with it this great big thing about polio and the epidemic. And it kept us abreast of what was going on, and it kept everybody very afraid. The pictures that went through my mind that night were the pictures of just rows upon rows upon rows of kids in wards in various stages of deformity and paralysis. Some in iron lungs, all of them in polio pants. That's something that I remember just so vividly, polio pants. They were like string bikinis. For various reasons they took pictures of

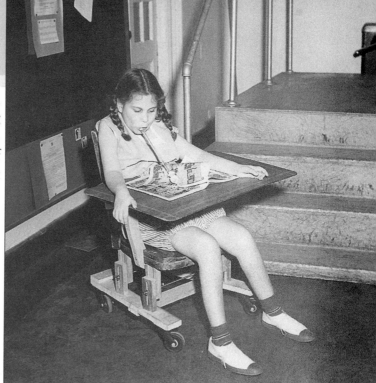

children without a whole lot of clothes on, I think to emphasize the crippling aspect of this disease. And so you would see the S-curve scoliosis on some of these children. I remember being very scared, very, very scared when I would go to the movies with my parents, through all those years before I was thirteen. Coming home from a movie probably two weeks before this happened, I remember asking my mother if that would ever happen to me. And she said. 'Charlene, I can't promise you that, but if we take good care of ourselves, if we don't go swimming in the late summer, if we don't go to all these places where strangers are, we take good care of ourselves and get plenty of rest...'

My first thoughts when the doctor told us were, 'I have polio, what's going to happen to me? Not only am I going to become this horribly crippled person, but who is going to want and like me?'

What happened when you got to the hospital?

Just prior to getting there, I pleaded with my mother not to leave me there. And I really didn't think she would. I had never been in a hospital for anything overnight, not even for tonsils. I remember my mother telling me how God was going to help me. I was confused about that. In fact, I wondered if I was being punished by God.

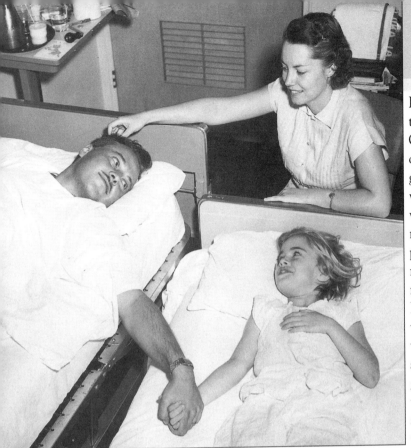

I learned very quickly, though, in the hospital, that God wasn't in the business of punishing me. When we got to the hospital they were waiting for me and came with a wheelchair. And I refused. I would not let them put me in the wheelchair. I remember my father telling me not to be so stubborn. But he also told me on the way to the hospital that I was made of good Finnish stick-to-it-iveness, and I was going to get through this. I was just going to have to be stubborn. So when I refused to get into that wheelchair, my parents and some aides came and helped me into the hospital. They got me into a chair right near the contagion unit door. I was in a ton of pain at that point. I heard somebody say that I had the stiffest back they had seen.

These doors swung open and my mother came to the door with me. And they said, 'You can't go beyond these doors.' And my mother said, 'I want to go with her.' And I remember crying, 'Mom, please don't leave me here.' And they just swung those doors. My mother's face was in this little window and she was crying. And my mother didn't cry frequently, and when I'd see my mother cry I knew things were serious. There were no parting, loving, kind words because they whisked me off so fast. And so I was crying really hard. And that was mixed with the pain. I remember just totally feeling alone in the world. And then I remember the sounds of that unit. There were iron lungs, and these iron lungs just pump and hiss and gush and pump and hiss and gush. And there were kids crying. The big city hospitals, Gillette and Sister

Kenny, all had big, huge wards. This was a contagion unit and I was whisked down this narrow hall into a room that really would have been a single, but they put two beds in it. And my bed was pushed up right against this window, looking out into the parking lot. I was absolutely terrified.

Your parents would come see you every day?

Not every day; they weren't allowed to come every day because it stressed me. They would have to stand outside my bedroom in the parking lot. The nurse would come over and open my window, not even an inch, just a tiny, tiny crack, so that we could hear. And I remember every day that they did come, my mother would insist that I raise my arms and I did. My arms weren't too terribly affected. And she'd tell me to lift my legs, and I did. But she wanted me to lift my head and I couldn't. And then one day my right leg didn't raise, no matter how hard I tried. And she started crying again. And she turned away and I remember feeling like I had let her down so bad. I was trying so hard to raise that leg and it didn't come up.

I remember my brother and cousins coming to see me. My brother's big, big eyes looking so scared at me. And then I remember the nurses telling me that they didn't think my parents should come too often because I became so emotional. It was hard for me, is what they thought. But I'll tell you what was hard: When my mother and dad would put their hands up on the window and I felt like I was in prison. And then she'd put her mouth over to the window and then blow me a kiss. This is a really, really lonely feeling. I knew they were cheering for me, praying for me, but I don't know that I have ever felt so alone.

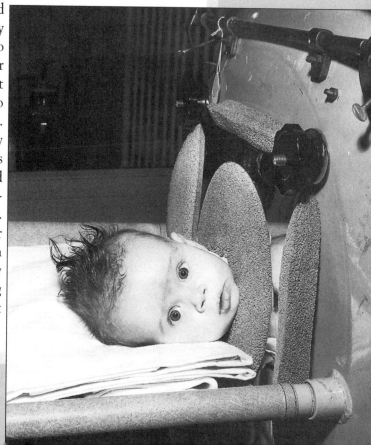

Tell me about what you saw and heard in the isolation unit.

That very same night I got there I ended up getting a roommate. I was very sick but this little girl seemed sicker. She was choking, gagging, crying. When they came in with her they raised the foot of her bed really high so that the phlegm would come out of her mouth. I remember the nurse turning her head, and kept turning her head to the side so she wouldn't choke. And I remember the horrid sound of her trying so hard to breathe and to swallow. And then I must have dozed off because I remember waking up and seeing her parents in the isolation room. And I asked the nurse why they can be in here and my parents can't. And the nurse said it was because they were short-staffed. They needed the parents to work this girl's throat muscles so she wouldn't choke. She was taken out that day and I never saw her again. I don't know if she ended up with a tracheotomy or if she was put in an iron lung.

What about some of the other people on the ward?

There was a boy that came in that night that was just terrifying to me. He came in and he was screaming and yelling and there was no room, so they put in a bed right outside of my door. He was in terrible pain and nothing was helping him. The next morning when he recognized that he was paralyzed he just screamed and yelled and flipped out of his mind. He was from Nashwack, Minnesota, and he had lettered in five sports. Five sports and he couldn't move below his neck. And I cried for him and prayed for him.

A pregnant woman came in a few days later. And the paralyzed boy was moved down the hall. They were still in the hall because there were no rooms. And this

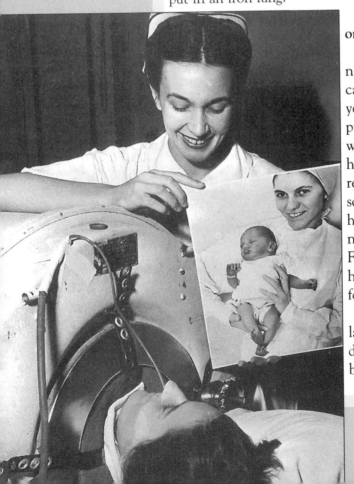

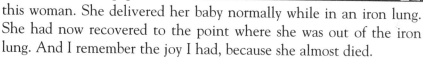

woman came in, in very bad shape and in a lot of pain. And I heard her doctor saying she is in crisis, this is a crisis. And he ordered an iron lung. And that sound stayed with me for years because that iron lung was right outside my door. They put her in that iron lung that night and then her husband was allowed to come into the unit because she was in a crisis stage, a critical stage. Years later my mother sent me an article from the paper about this woman. She delivered her baby normally while in an iron lung. She had now recovered to the point where she was out of the iron lung. And I remember the joy I had, because she almost died.

I remember the steamer kettles for the hot packs. There would be one layer, wet wool, and then they would come with this thick, heavy plastic piece that was cut the same shape and they'd put that over it. And then another piece cut the same shape out of dry wool. And then this was all pinned together. The packs had a very distinct sound and smell. Now, I don't think all hospitals had this, but I know that in Hibbing these hot pack steamer kettles smelled like wintergreen. They put wintergreen in them. If I passed wintergreen now I would be in that contagion unit in Hibbing. These kettles were round and they'd wheel them in. I had one put on my back. I loved the feeling because it was a comforting feeling. I mean it eased the pain, it helped. But I hated getting the packs put on because they had to move me and that hurt.

So that very first night they put this around me for my back. It covered my full torso, from my back to my bottom. And then another one around my neck and my thighs and my legs. And I felt I was being mummified, because then my feet were flat against a foot board at the end of the bed. I was left in those packs almost two hours. I was cold and they were itching, and I couldn't do anything about it. I remember deciding that if didn't complain I could get out of there fast. If I complained I'm going to be there longer.

Tell me what happened to your family while you were in isolation.

Well, my siblings and family were quarantined for two weeks. My father was a miner, and he was allowed to go to work because he was our provider. But miners came up from the mine, and they all would take a shower and leave their mining clothes at the mine. My father also had to take a shower as soon as he got to the mine, leave his street clothes in a bag, so as not to infect other men before he put on his mining clothes. It was that shower before going down that made him feel like he was separated. And he didn't mind doing that. It was a communicable disease.

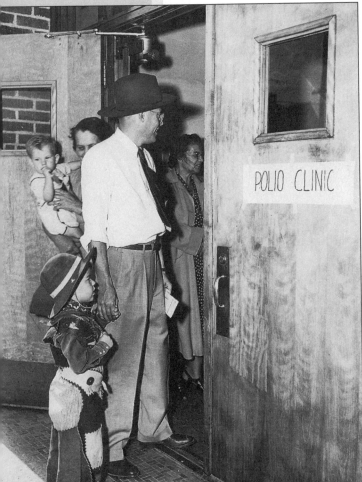

The school called to tell my parents that everything I had in my locker was gone. They had burned them. And they had burned my desk and they had burned all my school books and they had fumigated my locker. And my mother told me years later how awful that made her feel. But I had my American history book home, and nobody got sick from that book.

What was the response of the community toward your family?

First of all, when word got out that I had polio, the parents of these ten girls absolutely panicked. They didn't know what they should do. My parents, my sister who had gone away to college, and my brother and two cousins all were given shots of gamma globulin. But there was a shortage of gamma globulin and therefore my whole community couldn't be given these shots. I remember the parents of these ten girls were very angry at the public health department. They felt their daughters needed to be inoculated, because they had been with me. And yet none of them got sick.

I did some research myself, and looking back at newspapers from that time I found two small articles about me, that I had polio and I had been taken to Hibbing General Hospital, and then one little progress report. That's all. There are a lot of articles in those papers about marching for the March of Dimes and the Sister Kenny Foundation, and getting money and what it was used for. But there was no connection that these groups have already helped one of our own families.

I found that really interesting, that they didn't say there is a family here. Because my family was helped almost a hundred percent by the March of Dimes. The National Foundation of Infantile Paralysis was there for me, for my mom and dad, for the surgeries, for the hospitalization, for everything. It seemed as though you could collect more dimes if you connected to the dot over here, this one child in our community who was sick. But there was a fear. And I noticed in these articles there is also this little statement by the local doctor saying, 'It is not thought that her condition is considered serious. And there is no reason for us to believe that other cases will develop, but watch and be cautious.' And so forth and so on. And so it was almost like we don't want to put too much light on this.

How long were you in isolation?

I got out of contagion after ten days. And I was taken to a polio ward. I had several roommates by this time. One was the girl that was choking. Another was a first-grade teacher. Her name was Lois. She had a slight case of polio, she could get out of bed and walk, but she was there for a few days. And she was encouraging me. I remember her

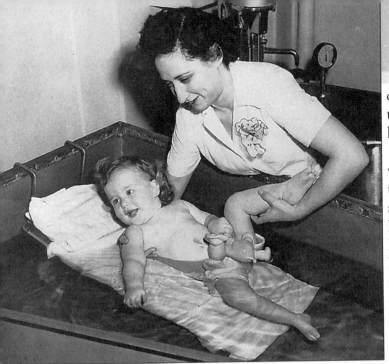

coming over to me and getting me to move my legs. And she would lift my legs, and try to lift my legs.

But most of the patients were younger than me: babies, two, three, four, five year olds. Those are the ones that took my heart. I hurt so bad for these children. Many little children of that age had polio in their faces. And their faces were becoming deformed and pulled out of shape. When children are too young, they don't understand how to work with therapy. They'd go to physical therapy, as I did, they'd get exercises, but they didn't go back to their rooms and practice opening and shutting their mouths. And they didn't want to do that either because it hurt the side of the muscles of the face that were affected. I really cared about these kids and I was ambulatory enough to visit them. Sometimes I used a chair, but otherwise I would use a railing in the hall. I remember one day asking my physical therapist, Marianne, if I could buy bubble gum for these kids. And she thought it was an excellent idea but she needed to clear it with the doctor in charge of each one of these kids. With facial paralysis there is also a chance of throat paralysis. Well, I got the clearance, as long as they didn't have paralyzed throats. And I got the gum and went to their rooms. I not only got them to chew but taught them to blow. By that push of the tongue it was using all these muscles and making their little tongues work.

Tell me about how you were finally able to leave.

I talked to my doctor and asked him if I could go home for a weekend. I'd been in the hospital for better than three weeks, almost four, which really isn't an inordinate amount of time for polio, but certainly was too long for me. And I asked him if I could go home for a weekend, and he said if the physical therapist said I was strong enough, and I would work on the muscle program while I was home, I could go home for the weekend. So I could call my parents to come and get me for the weekend, which I did. And my mother was very upset and believed that I was manipulating. So she called the doctor. And it hurt me terribly, it hurt me terribly because she said, 'No, we're not coming to get you. You're better off there. They're helping you. We're not coming to get you.' And it hurt me very, very bad because they didn't want to come get me. My parents called the doctor, who said I could go home for the weekend. By the time they got there I was going home for good. By this time my mother had already decided she was going to become my therapist, and she was learning the routine.

So when you went home, your mother acted as your therapist?

Yes, and prevented me from going to the Gillette Crippled Children's Hospital. I consider what my parents did for me, and they're both gone now, but I really consider what they did very heroic because they fought this disease with every fiber, and still raised other children and worked with me. My father would buy lead fishing weights, big, huge weights and other kinds of lead weights to make weights for my legs in my therapy routine. And the stretching exercises my mother would do, the hot baths at home, so hot that my body would be really red when I'd get out of there, but something about the sensation of that felt wonderful.

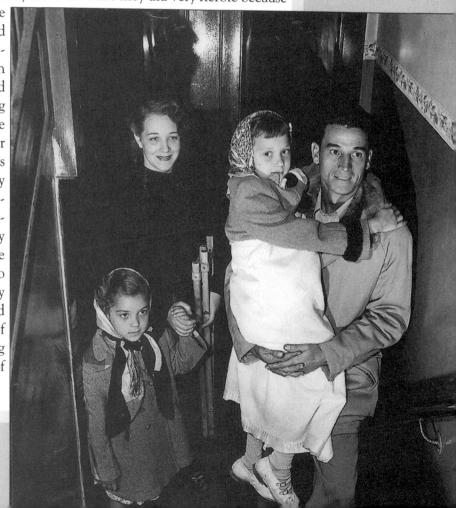

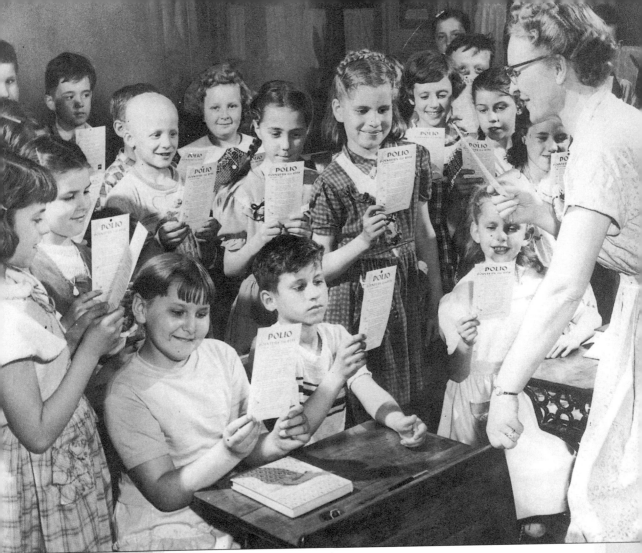

What about your friends?

My friends stayed away for quite a while. They called when I got home, but they stayed away. I guess what I felt at that time was it's because they were being told to. I don't think they were fearful I was contagious anymore. I believe that what they were concerned about was over-tiring me. As a polio survivor, or patient yet, I was required to nap in the morning and in the afternoon, and I needed to go to bed at eight o'clock at night. There was no school for me yet, so therefore if kids came over after school, it had to be very limited.

And what about when you went back to school?

Even before I got back the teachers started sending work home for me. They worked together really hard, they canceled a lot of assignments, a lot of stuff they didn't feel I had to do. When I went back to school, I never could take phys. ed. I felt unusual because of that. Being in school again, I remember being very determined that none of this was going to bother me. And what's interesting is that I went back to school right after Christmas and, in January, I formed a Junior Luther League in my church, so I guess I was very busy. I didn't just let things go by. I decided I've taken time off here, I didn't want to get left behind. I had a big fear of not finishing school with my classmates. I think it also helped me to be a determined person. That if I'm going to get anywhere in this world, if I'm going to walk, if I'm going to be disease-free, if I'm gonna do anything, I have to do something. I remember these thoughts in the hospital. I told my parents to bring me shorts and a shirt and a rug so I could practice physical therapy in my room between physical therapy sessions.

How did you feel when the polio vaccine was discovered?

My first reaction was almost anger. But it was selfish anger. It was anger that it didn't happen sooner, because in 1953 Dr. Salk was already conducting some trials, in 1954 more trials were conducted, and then I remember in 1955, when these big headlines came out. For me it was too little, too late. But I was so grateful that no one else would have to go through this. It was really something to celebrate. My children received the vaccine. I personally felt like I was an exclamation mark at the end of a headline screaming for the vaccine because having polio in 1953 and having the vaccine come out in 1954 was like, 'Wow, there I am, there's my exclamation mark,' that was my place in history. I remember my parents being very, very excited because no one would get it in my family again. And I'm really grateful to God that I am walking.

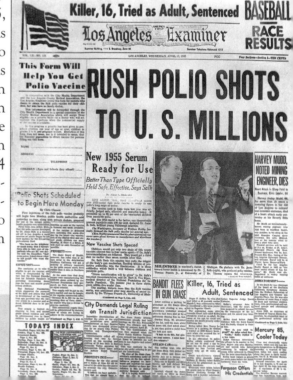

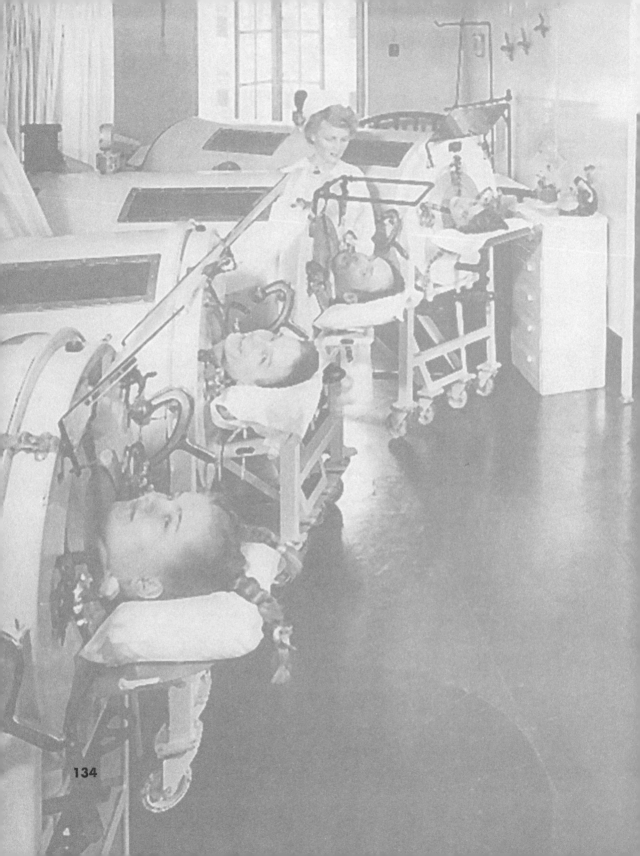

John Affeldt, M.D.

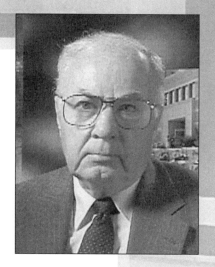

Dr. John Affeldt was a resident in internal medicine at Los Angeles County Hospital during the 1948 and 1949 epidemics. He later became the head of Rancho Los Amigos, one of the largest respiration centers for polio patients.

You were in residency in internal medicine in Los Angeles in 1948 and 1949, in the midst of a polio epidemic. What are your memories of that experience?

The communicable disease unit was a separate hospital at Los Angeles County Hospital and was built to receive cases of all infectious diseases, whether it be meningitis, typhoid fever, all kinds of very acute illnesses. So almost all of the acute polio patients that occurred in the Los Angeles area came to that hospital. I was in my residency at the White Memorial Hospital, which was about a mile away. And they called and said, 'Hey, we need help. We need more medical hands.' So they assigned me over there in the midst of the epidemic to help out. As such, I spent a year or so doing that, then I became chief resident. My day would be admitting acutely ill patients. They had probably gone to some other hospital or physician's office complaining of their illness and the physician thought, 'Hey, this might be polio.' So he just sent him or her over. And the ambulance would arrive. Then I'd get the report on it, check the symptoms, do the spinal tap, confirm the diagnosis: 'Yes, we do believe this to be polio.' And the symptoms would develop within hours, within days. They move quite rapidly. It wasn't necessarily everything going. It would be a little bit here, a little bit there, and you'd watch it: swallowing problems, if they found they couldn't breathe very well, couldn't move their arms or legs.

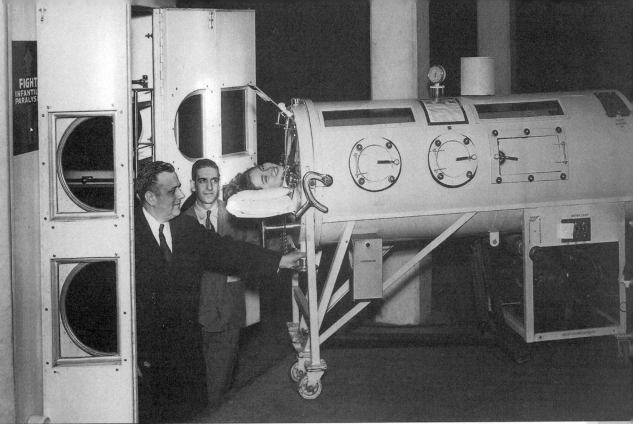

How many patients would come in during the epidemics?

The epidemics, of course, were primarily during the summer, not so much during the winter. Why, we don't know. So as the warm weather would come, we'd start receiving five to seven to ten patients per day. Some would clear up rather quickly. There was just no way of knowing how much paralysis, or lack of paralysis, or when the paralysis would disappear. Some would be discharged to other hospitals or programs to bring back functions.

How did you determine whether they needed to be in an iron lung?

If we had found that they were having trouble swallowing, mucus was accumulating, or they were choking, we'd have to call the throat surgeons over and they'd do the tracheotomy. We'd be measuring their respiration, how deeply they could breathe, checking the abdominal muscles, the diaphragm muscles, the chest muscles, the weakness occurring, the respiration dropping off. Then we put them in a respirator, get them accustomed to it, so they could breathe with it. The

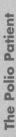

nursing staff knew how to teach them to relax, to go with it, instead of fighting it: 'Let it do it for you.' Finally, they learned how and found that their panic would diminish a little bit. Then 'Sister Kenny' hot packs would be applied. There was no treatment other than supporting respiration, swallowing food and water, and the hot packs. And, of course the family standing nearby in white gowns and masks would be frightened. They couldn't touch anything in that place. We were always afraid of germs and infectious diseases spreading, because we had chicken pox, measles, and whooping cough. And all these things mixed together was filthy.

Can you just sort of give me your mind's-eye image of the polio wards?

The acute polio wards, where the new cases came in, were in an old building. There were big, open wards, maybe only one or two private rooms for some of the worst infectious diseases. And of course there was always the noise of the respirators: whoosh...whoosh...whoosh. The sound of the machines for suctioning. Those that had tracheotomies would develop phlegm in their mouths—more like a gurgling sound, I guess. And I remember the sight of the physical therapists and the nurses coming around trying to position arms and legs.

What was the daily routine when you'd get an acute patient into the hospital?

After they are put into a bed or a respirator, depending upon the situation, from there on it's nursing care: bathing, feeding, trying to sleep at night. Those with paralysis, their noses would itch and somebody would have to come scratch it for them. You forget about those little things that we take for granted. They couldn't scratch. So they'd plead, 'Oh, please come scratch my face.' The little children, of course,

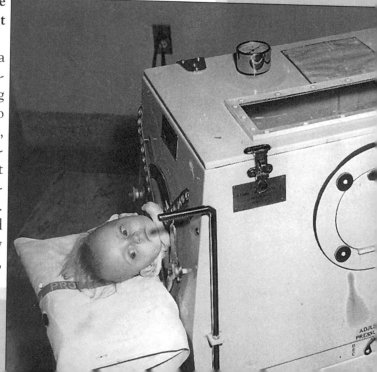

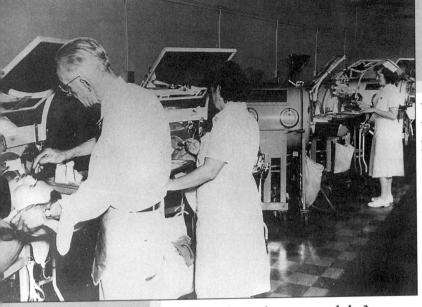

were very frightened. They were separated from their parents, brothers, and sisters. They would be put in a crib, crying. And finally cried themselves to sleep. The nurses and the therapists would come to work with them, try to distract them, try to get them to relax, if they could.

What about the young adults?

Well, for example, the twenty-five-year-old woman, the thirty-year-old woman, pregnant, would come in worried. We'd bring her obstetricians in to check them out and follow the progress, and to build muscle strength to deliver with. It really became quite an event, when labor would start and we would deliver the baby to a paralyzed mother. With a successful delivery, the staff was excited that they could manage to deliver to a woman that is paralyzed. The father would come in, the [other] children would come in, but they couldn't touch her. It was emotional.

Tell me about some of the special rules and rituals of the ward.

You could not touch the floor. If you dropped a pen, you could not pick it up. It was very common for the ladies to come in and sit down in the chair and put their purse on the floor and everybody would jump, 'Don't touch it.' They were not allowed to pick it up. Somebody would have to pick it up, clean it, to prevent infection. A piece of paper: everybody would reach to pick up. 'Oh, no, stop. Mustn't do that.' They later built another CD [communicable disease] unit, and the architects designed it so that the patient rooms had an outside passageway where the families could stand and look through the window at the loved one who was ill with an infectious disease.

Was it difficult to find nurses to work in these wards?

No, no, they were not afraid of it. Nurses, physicians, social workers, psychologists, attendants, food dispensers, nobody was afraid of it. Why, I don't know. And I don't really remember anybody working there becoming ill from it. I've often wondered why. Dealing with the height of the infectiousness of the disease, my assumption is that we were exposed through this process and we developed an immunity. Of course we protected ourselves with gloves and gowns and masks, but it's airborne. Into your mouth and you've got it. So we must have had some immunity. But somehow or other you're not afraid of it.

What do you remember about the fear of the general public?

In those days, when the epidemic started sweeping through Los Angeles they closed the theaters, they closed the swimming pools, they stopped having get-togethers. They stopped doing tonsillectomies, because it seemed that the person who had recently had a tonsillectomy was more apt to get the bulbous type of polio. Folks were afraid to go to school. It's hard to realize that today, when we don't have an epidemic like that anymore.

Why don't we talk a little about the story of Rancho Los Amigos?

The communicable disease unit [at Los Angeles County] could hold only so many patients, so when the acute polios kept coming, seven, ten a day into respirators, they had to relieve that pressure and move them out. So that's when they started transporting them to Rancho, which became sort of a storage area. That sounds awful, but basically that's what it was. Because there was little or no therapeutic or rehabilitation program there, they were sent there to relieve the pressure of the new ones coming in. And so they were housed in the respirators at Rancho, and the numbers grew. They got up to about one hundred or so respirators, and Rancho was not equipped to do this. The families would get together, and they were real concerned that there

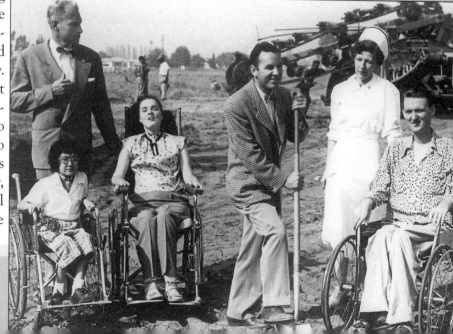

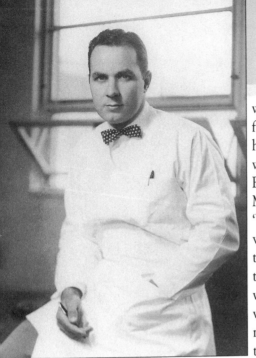

was not a real active program to try to restore some function to the patients. They had meetings, and somehow or other Drew Pearson got hold of the story and was about to make a national scandal out of the story of Rancho. So the County of Los Angeles turned to the March of Dimes and the Polio Foundation and said, 'We need help.' The March of Dimes turned to Harvard, where I happened to be doing research on respiration, which came from my polio days in Los Angeles. So they tagged me. A nurse from New York and myself went and spent two weeks studying the problems and we made a report. They had a meeting and they called me in and said, 'Well, you made these recommendations, why don't you go do it?'

And what did you find, when you got there?

Wards full of respirators and a very dedicated nursing staff, but no knowledge as to how to proceed. There was an elderly nurse in a cubicle with a microphone. They called her 'Gravel Greet' because she would get on the microphone to say things to the patients. When I came we started developing our research laboratory—how to do better measurements of the respiration, how to know how they were doing, how can we get them out of the respirators?

Rancho was originally the county pig farm. There were cows, horses, growing fields, vegetables. So when the respirator patients were sent in, they took over some old buildings. And they were pretty drab. As I said, it was a warehouse of patients. It was a custodial program. There was no hope. When I came in, the staff was very skeptical of my ability to do anything different than they were doing. The key test was when the rocking bed arrived, and I said, 'We're going to get a patient out of the respirator here.' And the staff gathered around with a look on their faces. 'You're going to fail, this patient's gonna die [if you take him out].' Real tension and anxiety. We took the patient out of the respirator, put him on the rocking bed, and he started rocking. The patient was breathing with the bed. And the patient became so animated. 'I can scratch my face! I can touch my nose!' The staff just

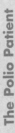

turned on. I mean it was a turning point. From then on, the staff couldn't move fast enough to start working on how to get the patients out of the respirators.

We were able to develop a device to measure the breathing so we could tell how long to keep them out of the respirator. Ten minutes, thirty minutes, two hours. We took them out of the machine so they could cough. And once you could get them out of the respirator part-time, then the chest respirators came along. So now they're in the bed free. You can get physical therapy and occupational therapy to them. You could start doing things that you couldn't in the respirator. One of the peculiar things that happened was that there were two competing companies: Emerson Company & the Huxley Company. And the Huxley engineer—a bright guy from the famous Huxley family—says

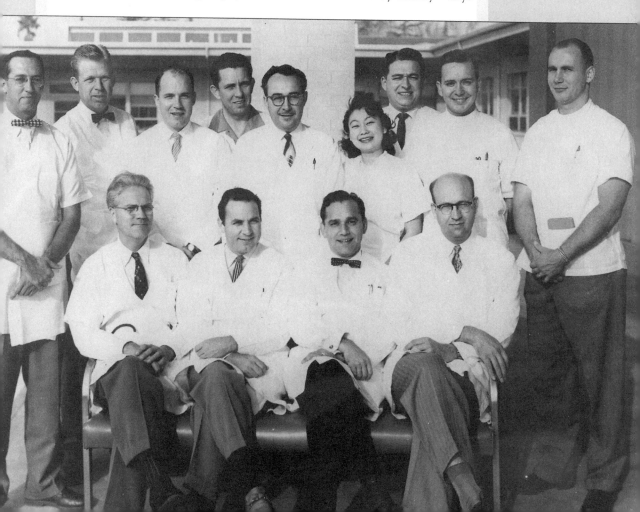

to me, 'How come every time the patients want to go home for the weekend, they take my Huxley off and they want an Emerson?' Well, we didn't know. Finally our psychologists, who were dealing with the patients, gave me the answer. The Huxley went way down under the body, including the abdomen. The Emerson was just the chest. The patients could have sexual relations with an Emerson. They couldn't in a Huxley. Strange story but true.

What kind of help did you have?

There was a lot of volunteer support—Hollywood support. Folks would come out and do things for the patients. They would donate money, donate devices. Everybody mobilized to raise the morale. As we'd get 'em out of respirators, we started making special braces and things that were mechanical to try to put functions back into the hand and the wrist and the elbow and the shoulder. In fact, this man McKibben, who helped devise the first atom bomb, his daughter was a patient there. And he came and said, 'How can we get some muscle function here?' So he devised a little rubber device with a Chinese finger trap. They could use their tongue or their lips or their forehead to trigger a valve and they'd get a pinch. You know how important that pinch is? You now have a function that you didn't have before. So it

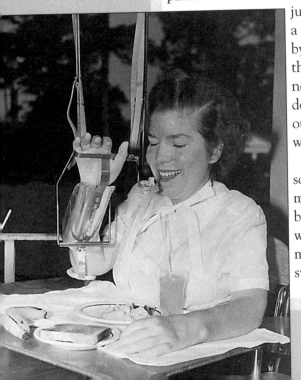

just moved on with developments. Then Rourke, a big defense manufacturer in San Diego, came by. His son was there in a respirator. I took him through the place and he said, 'What do you need?' I said we need money to develop these devices. And he gave us stock. Out of that came our bioengineering department, which came up with major developments.

One of our key staff physicians noticed that some of our patients had peculiar swallowing mechanisms that seemed to enable them to breathe. He observed and finally realized that what they were doing was swallowing air as a means of breathing. He took x-ray films of the swallowing and he called it glossular pharyngeal breathing. He also called it frog breathing because they were gulping like a frog. So he learned how to do it himself, and he taught his staff how to do it. Then he taught patients how to do it, and it became a very major development of freeing patients from the respirator. They couldn't do that in their sleep, but it was a wonderful safety mechanism for those who could be out of the respirator for x number of hours.

How did patients handle that weaning process from the respirators?

The patients wanted out. There was fear, yes. They had to be reassured that staff was there to help. And so the weaning process was measuring their ability to breathe. When would they get tired? When would they have to go back in the respirator? How long could they stay out? What could they do while they were out? And then of course there were exercises for the diaphragm, for the chest muscles. A positive pressure device was put on the mouth or the tracheotomy to support them. And it worked.

Were there any educational or social programs?

There were always attempts at social programs, entertainment, reading. For the children we had school teachers who would come and give them classes. We had a schoolroom, for those we could get into wheelchairs. But if they were in a respirator, it had to be done at the site of the respirator. For the adults there was television. Somebody had donated enough television sets so that every ward had one. One of the social programs that emerged and was [based on] the Miss America beauty pageant. The program director and the patients' families cooked up this idea of a beauty queen. 'Miss Breathless,' they called it—who was the prettiest lady in a respirator? And so the volunteers would come in and fix them up. They would prepare for this for a long time. And they would have ballots and finally we'd gather the respirators out in the patio in the circle there and announce the winner. One of those years when we had the Miss Breathless contest Ronald Reagan and Nancy came out from Hollywood and crowned Miss Breathless. A great event for the patients.

How did the children handle paralysis?

Some of the children really impressed me. I thought about it many times over the years. They had paralysis of the upper extremities, but their legs were not paralyzed and they learned to use their toes like hands. I mean they were so adept. I'd walk up to the bed, their foot would reach down. They'd pull a pistol out of the holster and point it at me and say, 'Bang! Bang!' This was now like their hands. And they learned to write, to do their school work with a pen, a pencil, feed themselves—amazing. I thought about this in terms of our society. Supposing we learned to use our feet young, like our hands. We would have four dexterous extremities instead of two. We would dress differently. We would sit differently. Our homes would be different. Our cars would be different. It would be a different society. But we'd never take advantage of that.

Do any particular patients stand out in your mind?

There was one lady who was severely paralyzed and ended up at Rancho and eventually got out of the respirator. The occupational 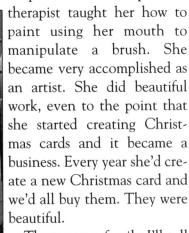 therapist taught her how to paint using her mouth to manipulate a brush. She became very accomplished as an artist. She did beautiful work, even to the point that she started creating Christmas cards and it became a business. Every year she'd create a new Christmas card and we'd all buy them. They were beautiful.

There was a family I'll tell you about—a very prominent

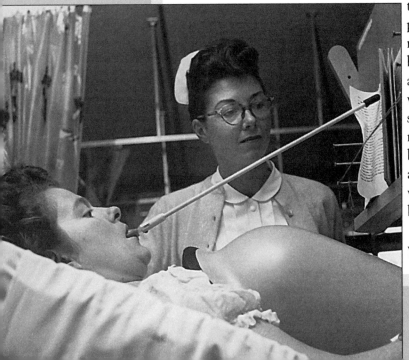

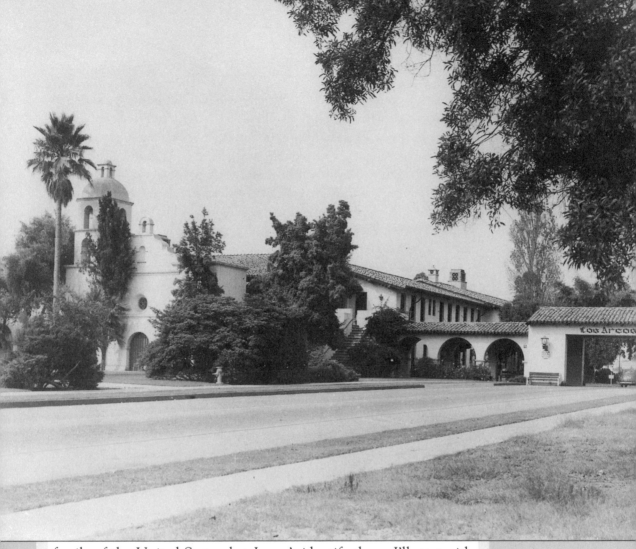

family of the United States, but I won't identify them. I'll start with the young boy, a teenager at the time. He was playing touch football with his brothers on the front lawn. And then all of a sudden he fell down. He had paralysis of the legs, we brought him in. I met with the father and the mother, and he ended up in the respirator for a short time but recovered from that and was in a wheelchair. He became a top national rehabilitation expert in the world. A little bit later, when the vaccine came along, his brother was in training as an Air Force pilot down in Texas. The first doses of vaccines were made available to the military there, and there were just enough doses to go around with one missing. So, as the captain of that crew, he made sure the vaccine

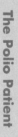

The Polio Patient

went to his crew and he didn't take any. A very short time after that he came down with polio and paralysis. They sent an Air Force jet to take me down to Texas to treat him and I can remember he was in the respirator, starting to have trouble swallowing and I said, 'You've got to have a tracheotomy.' And he was devastated. Here was his pilot's helmet hanging at the side of the respirator. He knew then that he would never fly again. We did the tracheotomy. He improved to the point where he got out of the respirator. He became ambulatory with crutches and canes.

Let's talk about the vaccine. What was the response from the patients and the families about the announcement that the Salk vaccine worked?

I attended the meeting in Ann Arbor, Michigan, where it was announced. We were delighted—elated. Back with the polio patients and the families, there was no resentment—'Why didn't they have it for me?' There was delight that epidemics would cease. The medical staff was delighted that they wouldn't have to go through these traumatic stressing times of more patients coming in, more disability and sorrow. It was a great thing. I was acquainted with both Sabin and Salk, and I remember a meeting where we were planning the International Polio Conference for Geneva, Switzerland. My wife and I would be at these meetings and we'd bump into Salk or Sabin in the back corridor one at a time, and each one tell us how their vaccine was better than the other.

Juanita Howell, R.N.

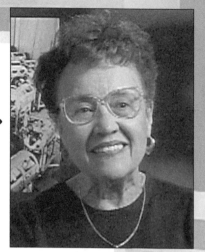

Juanita Howell was a polio nurse during the big epidemic in Mississippi in 1946. In 1948 she was one of three African-American nurses who went to study the Sister Kenny treatment for rehabilitating muscles paralyzed by polio.

How did you come to be a polio nurse?

I was working in Mississippi in 1946 and we had an epidemic there. I was a school nurse and we were closing down for school, so I was without employment. Although in those days nurses could walk across the street and get another job, I thought, well, why don't I try the polio clinic? They were advertising for help. They needed help, the patients were coming from all around the state, nurses were coming from all over the country, it was just a very desperate time. It was just one of those very dramatic times in history, I guess. By not having a family, I could do this. I could go to work at four in the afternoon, I could go at eleven o'clock at night. We had a lot of nurses who came back from the war in 1945, and they followed the epidemics. Probably because they were available.

Describe your average day in Jackson, Mississippi, in 1946.

We went to the hospital in our street clothes, because we were concerned about the average citizen's reaction to us catching the bus where they knew the polio clinic was, and getting on with our uniforms. So they advised us to wear our street clothes. They had an area right inside the door where we changed into a kind of scrub-gown thing. And we went in and did what we needed to do to, help these people. We would wipe their tears, we would wipe drool, we fed them, we brushed their hair, we bathed them, we took care of body eliminations, everything. We'd move their fingers, position their hands—

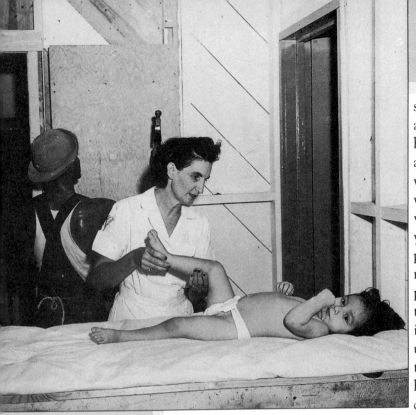

some of them were paralyzed and could not move their hands. And you had to be aware that this little finger was not tucked under an area where pressure would develop on it. The last thing you wanted was for this patient, who already had so many problems, to develop a pressure sore. We changed their positions, we put cushions between their knees, under their heels. We tried to put hot packs on them, we had some in iron lungs, depending on where you worked for the day. It was a large room, and we tried to have the machines situated so there was space between them, so that the bellows could move back and forward without hitting the walls. The patients' heads were all positioned to the center of the room, so that the nurses standing in the center of the room could catch a look at each patient. Oftentimes they could not get your attention vocally. You had to be aware and alert all the time. It was that kind of thing, just kind of common sense, doing what was necessary to make a person feel comfortable. There was no medication. There was no proven anything at that point in time.

How did you bathe them?

Well, we would have a pan of water and we'd bring out our towel. The iron lung had access. You'd open it like a port hole on a ship and put your arm in. With your arm in there, there was a kind of foam rubber that sealed it so that you didn't break the air pressure. And you'd get the other arm in there and wipe them off. Maybe it took so much longer than it would have for an ordinary bed bath, but we did what we could.

Tell me about dealing with their emotional trouble.

Well, it was a trust thing. Just like any other illness, if a patient got the idea that you were going to do the best you could for them, then they let you and didn't create a problem about it. I think that was one of the things that I experienced. I had a good rapport with my patients.

Can you describe those patients who were hardly visited?

It's kind of awesome when I think of it now, that we had those children seven days a week and their parents came on Sunday afternoon and that was it. And it was accepted by the children and it was accepted by the parents. It was like, well, that's the way it is and everyone went along with it. I think we would not get away with that now, they would have you in court or something if you tried it. But that's the way it was.

How did you feel about the little children?

It was kind of tragic because the little children bonded with the people who were taking care of them. You would take care of this kid all week long, and then on Sunday, when mother came to visit, oftentimes they became closer to you than mother, which was very hard for her and a little embarrassing for you. You thought, they're thinking that I've been brainwashing this child or trying to take their place. But it was just a human thing that happened. You would have to be careful when the parents came to visit that you were able to make that transfer, get the child to his parents without him wanting to hang on to you or come back to you. That initial transfer was always a little bit traumatic. A lot of times patients would [confuse] the caring and professional environment [with] a lasting affection. And that was not necessarily what was on the professional's mind.

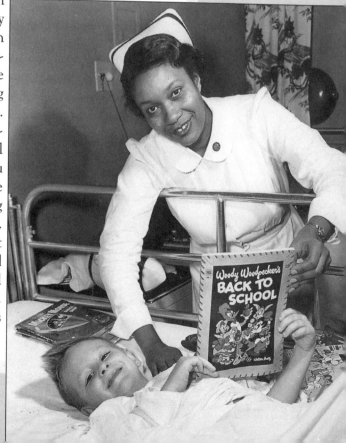

What about the older children?

The older children and the young adults couldn't wait for the weekend. They talked about their mothers and dads coming and they would be bringing presents and things, so it would be better for them. And the hospital provided the schools for these children. I think being ill and being lumped in with different ages of children did have a maturing effect on them. They had no real playtime, you see. They spent their time getting treatments, going to their classes, and some of them had an insight that was remarkable for little children. Oftentimes I would just look at them when they would tell me things and think, 'Wow.' I think it was because of the environment they were in. They didn't get to go outside or play, they were in that hospital twenty-four hours a day.

Did you have a feeling of desperation or hopelessness for some of these children?

Not desperation, but I knew they were going to die, if that's what you mean. But I think this is what nursing is really all about. You're fighting a battle that you know you're not going to win. But you keep doing the best that you can for the time that you have.

Can you talk about the progress of patients and weaning someone from an iron lung?

The iron lung was a bed that would roll out. You start out by just opening the machine so that the pressure was off for as long as they could

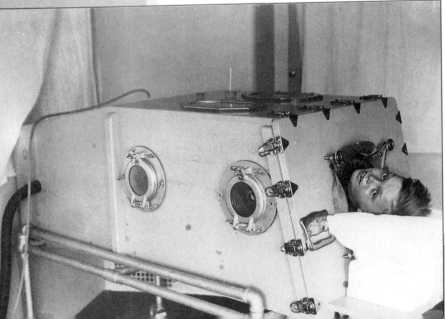

breathe a little bit on their own. Sometimes it was twenty minutes, sometimes it was longer and it gradually got better. And then they would go from there to the rocking bed and all the time new things were being developed. There was another breathing device; I

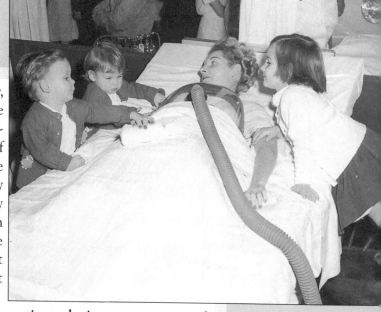

don't know the name of it right now, but it just fit over the chest and the air pressure was attached like a floor-type vacuum cleaner. I don't know if it was psychological, but a lot of the patients were afraid of it. They wouldn't want to sleep in it, they would want to go back to the iron lung to go to sleep. [They were afraid] of not being able to get enough air, because this was what it did. It breathed for them.

What happened to the iron lung patients during a power outage?

Some hospitals had generators that we used during outages. In Mississippi there was a lot of weather that played havoc with the regular electricity, so that was provided, but that wasn't enough and until they got the generators operating, someone had to provide the manual power. The machines could be switched into manual and operated by hand. There was a crank on the back of it, and maintenance people, gardeners, sweepers, anybody who was available, came to help do that.

Describe your work during the big polio epidemics.

When the polio epidemic quieted down in Mississippi, I thought it was time to do something else. So I went to Evanston, Illinois, and worked in a community hospital doing general-duty nursing. And all that time that I was there I would hear on the radio requests for nurses to come to Minnesota and take the program from Sister Kenny. I kept thinking about it and one day I just picked up the phone and applied to the National Institution of Infantile Paralysis for a scholarship to come and learn Sister Kenny's treatment for polio patients. I got married in 1950 and had two little children over the next two years and didn't work. In 1953 there was a big epidemic year and they needed help, so they called me and I worked the 3:00 to 11:30 shift. I went there after my husband came home from work and he was with the children while I was at Sister Kenny. And then he'd leave the children asleep and run to the institute to pick me up around 11:30.

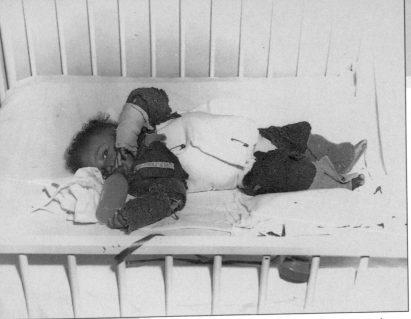

Did you ever fear bringing polio back to your own children?

You know that's a strange thing, but I did not. I'm sure I would not have done it if I would have any idea that it might happen to them.

Can you tell me about the hot packing, especially in the summer?

The hot packing was a comforting thing for the patient. These packs where heated in big vats of boiling water. They were moved from the vat to a machine that extracted all of the water because any water left in the pack could burn the skin. But the hot pack was a comfort for the skin and the muscle. But those people who applied these hot packs, well, we would perspire to the point where our clothes stuck to us.

How did you feel when the vaccine came out?

I said, 'Yes!' I was thrilled. It was a wonderful thing, a marvel, a godsend that this terrible disease was finally done with. And the people who worked with it were able to transfer their skills. It didn't put anybody out of work. Polio was a terrible scourge on our country for the time, but people died from other things too.

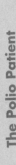

The Polio Patient

Clara Yelder

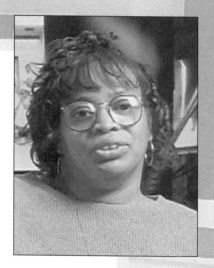

Clara Yelder lived in the rural community of Prattville, Alabama, when she contracted polio at the age of six. Because medical facilities in the South were segregated, she could not be treated in local hospitals, so she stayed at the all-black Infantile Paralysis Center at Tuskegee Institute for her year and a half of therapy and rehabilitation.

What's your first memory of polio?

I was six years old and all I can remember is I was at a clinic, there were lights, my dad was crying. I don't remember how I got there. I don't know why I was there. All I know was that I was there and dad was crying. I know my mother was there but she was more reserved, more quiet. The doctor was saying, 'No, you can't take her home.' And that's when I realized that something was wrong. It just all happened so fast, it was all so strange.

Tell me a little bit about your family and about where you lived.

I have a very large family. At that time I had six or seven sisters and brothers. We lived in a poor, very rural area. There were probably three black families—one happened to be my grandparents—and perhaps twenty white families. My father was a janitor, my mother was a housewife. We didn't have a car or a phone. My grandparents had a phone. And for black people it was like the phone booth—everybody used their phone. So my parents called someone who had a car and hired them to take us to the hospital.

Tell me about the hospital.

Well, they took me straight to Tuskegee after the initial examination. I remember Dr. Kaiser saying, 'No, you can't take her home, she

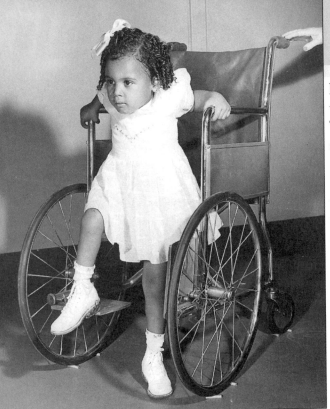

has to go straight to Tuskegee.' That's where they took the black polio victims. The white kids were sent to Warm Springs and other areas.

What happened at Tuskegee?

I remember the first two weeks there I was in isolation, so I didn't see any of my family. The first two weeks the only memory I have of my family is just their heads sticking through the door. It was so quiet, and all you saw were eyes, because when the attendant staff came in they were masked and gowned. So it was like a different world. It was very quiet. And I think that when I was awake, I cried constantly. My parents could only come up on Sundays, and they would have to take turns because there were small kids [at home]. So it was only twenty minutes away, but I might as well have been in another state.

I was in Tuskegee for at least a year and a half. The walls were very light green. There probably were from six to eight beds to a ward, and they were always just about filled. As I can remember, there were mostly girls. They were around the age I was. And I made some long-lasting friends. But I missed my home so much. I mean, they were going on with their life without me. But I was one of the lucky ones. My parents did come to see me once a week, and most of the kids' parents never did. I don't know whether they were from farther away than I, were poorer than I, but they never had visitors. I remember there were very few.

Besides treatments, how did you pass the time?

We talked. And eventually we had a radio. The center of our day was listening to the radio. There were no televisions. When I got to be in a wheelchair, we used to have wheelchair races. It was a very slow race. And when our birthdays came around, they always gave us a gift. We were allowed to go outside. I used to remember watching the ROTC at Tuskegee. On Sunday morning when they used to drill, that was fun.

As a six-year-old, did you know you would never walk again?

When I saw the other kids fitted with their braces and long crutches, I knew the same thing would probably happen to me. I had resigned myself that I wasn't going to walk again. Well, I guess like anybody I had dreams that someday I would walk out of there. Only dreams. I mean, when I woke up, when daylight reality hit, the dreams stopped.

Were there any iron lungs in your ward?

I remember this particular girl. We got to be friends. All I ever saw was her head. I learned later what would have happened to her if she hadn't been in there, but at that time it was very strange.

You were also in the Montgomery Clinic. Tell me about that.

The white and the black children were on the same floor there but we were divided. The white kids were way down the hall and it was like another world. I don't know what went on in their section. In our section, I was in a room with two beds. Sometimes they did sneak two more in there.

What happened when you learned you were going to go home?

I was fitted with my braces and I actually got up on crutches. And even though I could only go a few paces, I guess they would say I was at the point that the rest of the treatment could be finished at home, so I was allowed to go home.

Oh, that was the biggest thrill. I thought it was all over. I thought I would never have to see a hospital again, never have to see another doctor again as long as I lived. I really thought that. At home, my grandparents were there, all my sisters and brother was there. It's something you can't describe. I was coming home. That's all I can say. I was home.

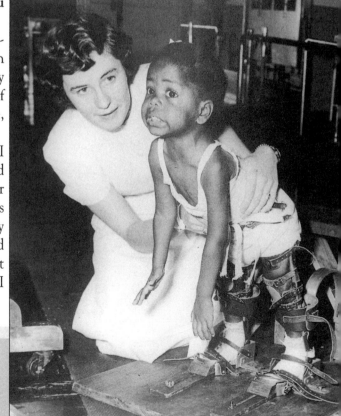

Did you get around in a wheelchair?

No, not at first. I suppose I didn't need one. Because it was a small house, one of my parents or older sister and brother would carry me every place I needed to go. And they would bring my dinner to me so I didn't have to go to the dinner table with the rest of the family. I was probably nine or ten when I got my first wheelchair. There was a man in my community, and his wife happened to name me when I was a baby. And he did a fundraiser and bought me a wheelchair. [Later] I was in the Miss Alabama Wheelchair contest. Well, it's not really a contest. It's an achievement program to let the public know what we're all about. It's not a beauty contest. Oh, that was fun. I came in third, or second runner up. I think it sounds better to say I was second runner up.

What was your relationship with the March of Dimes?

I know the March of Dimes must have helped me a lot because every year, I remember my dad marched for the March of Dimes. He never missed marching. Never.

Tell me about your schooling.

When I got back home, my dad went to the superintendent of education, and he said, 'no,' they would not take the responsibility of me attending public school. And that was it. So I stayed home with my mom. So when the other kids went off to school I did nothing.

Eventually you did get an education. Tell me about that.

Eventually, yes. It was mostly done on my own. I would read the books that my sisters and brothers read. I would read their homework, I would read everything I could get my hands on. And eventually I started taking some night classes. One of my sisters' teacher, out of the kindness of her heart, decided she would come out at least once a week and go over homework with me. So a few years later, I went to rehab for about eleven months and I got a GED. I was twenty-nine when I got the GED. It took me another couple of years to make up my mind to go to college [for a degree in history]. Oh, those were the fun years. I went to Troy State, here in Montgomery. At Troy State, they were great. For a few classes I had friends that would put me in class. But then I told someone there, and they built portable ramps. So they adapted the campus to me.

John Hume, M.D.

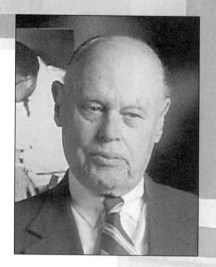

Dr. John Hume went to Alabama to head the orthopedic surgery unit at Tuskegee University beginning in 1949. He was the only certified black orthopedic surgeon in the South. Except for the white bracemaker, the entire staff at the Polio Unit at Tuskegee, run by Dr. Hume, was black and it provided the only polio services for black children in the South.

Tell me about Tuskegee and its role with polio in the South, going back before you came there in 1949.

In the epidemic period of 1936, the epidemic among blacks in the South was something new, because most polio cases were either in New England or in the Midwest. At that time, there was no place in America that had the complete facilities to treat blacks, such as they had at Warm Springs. So the problem was that all these hospitals were segregated. The blacks were put in separate waiting rooms and had to wait 'til all the white patients were seen. Or they put them in the basement, and then had to have the parents nurse them. So what are you going to do with these children who are seriously ill, who need specialized care? And in some instances need an iron lung, and even surgery. Well, you understand that a preacher from Mobile had a son who had polio, and he wanted to get him admitted to Warm Springs. Well, Warm Springs turned him down. Warms Springs is in the middle of Georgia and the rules of segregation in those times prohibited the admission and treatment of black patients. In the meantime, President Roosevelt had developed the March of Dimes program. And blacks were contributing. Things got so bad that the black newspapers, the NAACP, President Roosevelt, Eleanor Roosevelt, Basil O'Connor, and all the rest of them

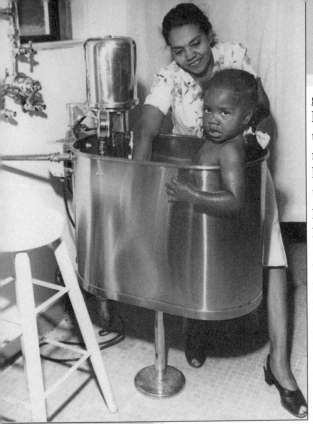

got together. Roosevelt and Mrs. President Roosevelt got on the officials at Warm Springs to do something about it. The bottom line was, no, we can't treat black patients because we'd have to build a new pool, a ward for them and that was expensive. The best thing would be to put a unit in an institution that treated black patients and had the necessary staff to handle it. And of course here in Tuskegee they had a well-known medical educational program, and we had clinical society meetings where renowned physicians came from all over the country and lectured and demonstrated the latest things to the black physicians.

Describe the makeup of the polio unit at Tuskegee.

This unit had thirty beds in it. We had pediatricians, we had nurses, an occupational therapist, physical therapist, and we had social workers. The only thing that was needed was bracing. They had a shoe shop over on campus here where the kids learned to mend shoes, and they did some brace work. But after a while we got a bracemaker to do the work. All of the staff were black except for the bracemaker. He had his business in Montgomery and he came to Tuskegee and took the measurements, made the braces, and he was the only white person on the staff.

What did the unit look like?

It had a glass room, treatment room, a physical therapy unit, which contained exercise equipment, an occupational therapy unit, where they made clay things and wove and so forth, and a therapeutic pool that was located in the basement. And up a floor it had Woolworth's.

Talk about epidemics in 1951 to 1952.

One thing you have to understand is that the polio disease had several courses. In the beginning polio was manifested by an upper respiratory infection, which lasted maybe three to four weeks and then there was a period following where you had intense muscle spasms and pain as a result of the paralytic process, and then finally we had to restore the muscles and put patients through physical therapy and occupational therapy. And of course one of the big problems were patients who required an iron lung in order to make it, and that was a big problem among the local people in Mississippi, Georgia, and Louisiana.

The biggest challenge was that children had to stay in the hospital from six months to two, three years, and people in the rural communities couldn't drive in here anytime and visit. So there were letters written by the mother and letters written by the sisters to the children, and the social worker answered these letters and was advising the family of the progress of their children. It was very difficult for the rural families. Another difficulty was continuing the education that was needed for these kids. They had two teachers who came into the unit and gave classes.

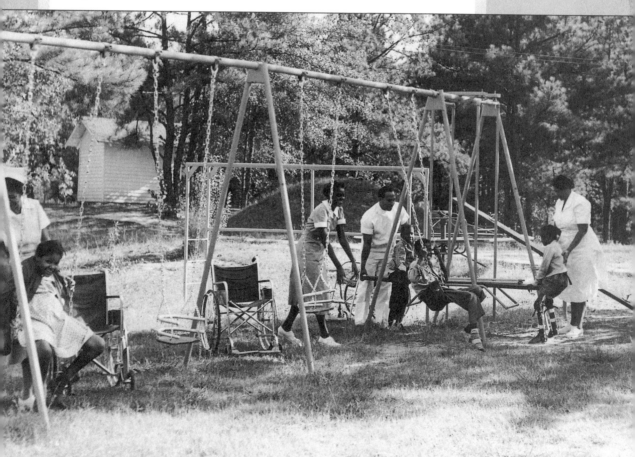

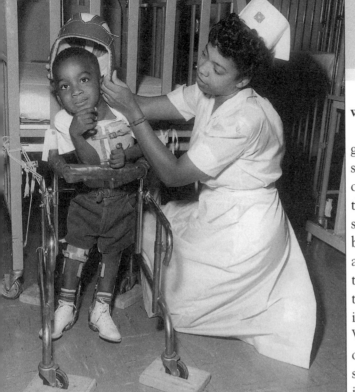

Tell me about your relationship with the doctors at Warm Springs.

In order to bring the treatment program up to date at our infantile paralysis unit, we went to Warm Springs and observed their work. And after that they came to Tuskegee and demonstrated operative procedures, and the brace man came from Warm Springs and showed us how they were bracing their patients. So it was a two-way thing, although we never were involved in treating any patients at Warm Springs. And when we began operating on our patients, the load started dropping because we were treating them and discharging them.

Was there any awkwardness about the interactions between the black and white doctors?

It was on a professional level and there was no indication that we were being patronized and there was no hostility toward us. They were quite taken with the operating facilities and there was typical, professional accord among blacks and whites and the color business didn't enter into our relationship. [However], when the staff of Tuskegee went to Warm Springs, at lunch time we were separated. And we just didn't buy it, we just didn't go along with the plan, and they became embarrassed and set up this table in the president's dining room.

How big an impact did Tuskegee have?

The problem with black care in the South was segregation, which existed within medical systems and hospitals and doctors' offices. So Tuskegee was an oasis for black medical care in the South. It was the only place where all of the necessary care was available to black children, so it had a big impact. And the work at the polio unit resulted in the training of black physical therapists and black occupational therapists, and it even informed physicians about the disease who were not orthopedists but general practitioners who came to Tuskegee for the clinical society meetings every year. You know, blacks were excluded from medical societies and from areas where they would be conducting medical education. But the crucial point about it is that all of the personnel who took care of these patients were black, and it proved that we could do the job.

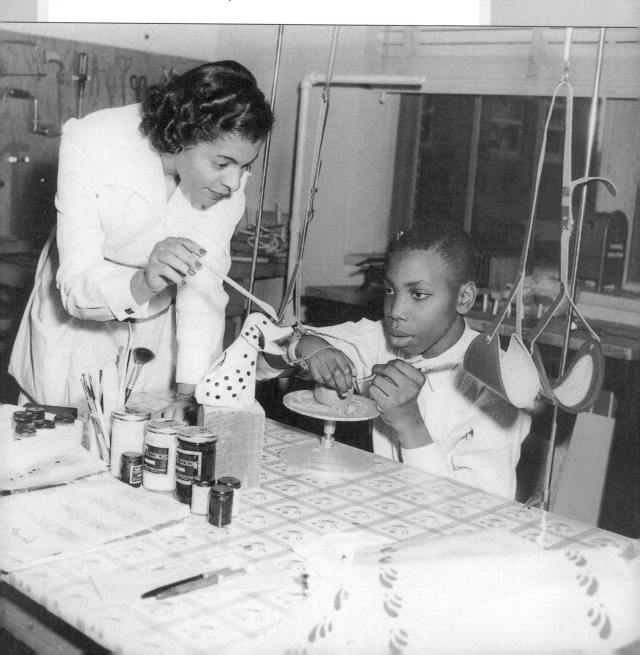

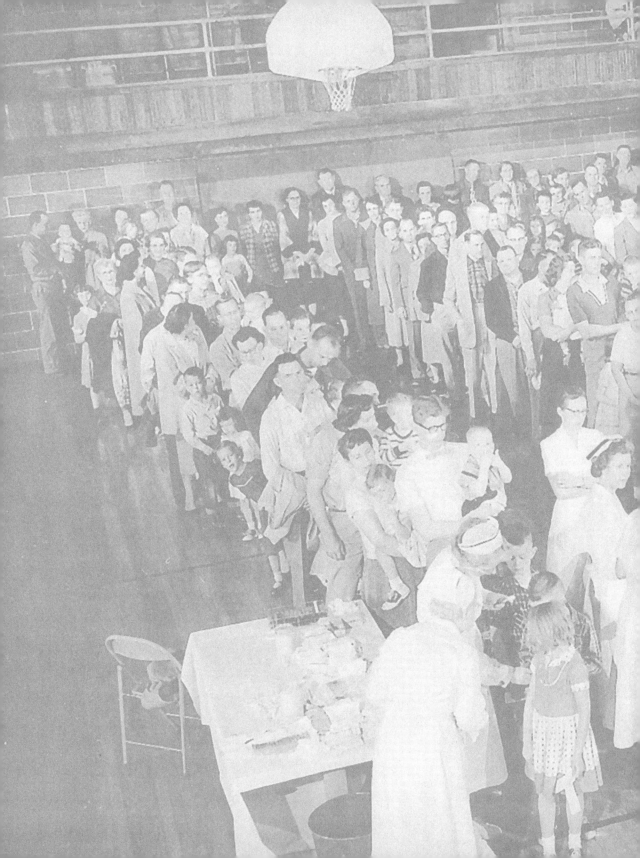

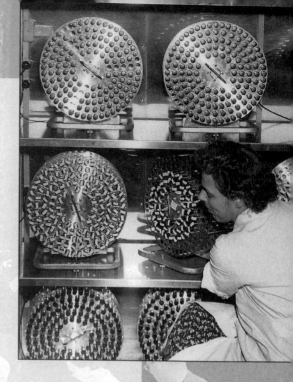

Chapter 5

Salk, Sabin, and the Search for a Vaccine

Jonas had the idea, from a time when he was quite young, that he wanted to do something that would make a difference to humanity. And so he was fueled by an idealism that was sincere, backed by all the scientific knowledge, and his personality, and his ability to follow through. It was extremely important to him to achieve and that's exactly what he did.

—Donna Salk,
first wife of Dr. Jonas Salk

Even before the New York epidemic of 1916, doctors had begun to research the causes and treatment of this puzzling new ailment. In the late nineteenth century, the German orthopedist Jacob Heine saw some of the earliest polio paralytics and provided basic clinical studies of the effects of the disease. Oskar Medin, studying a Swedish epidemic of 1905, realized that polio was an infectious disease. Ivar Winkman, another Swede, suggested that the disease was spread

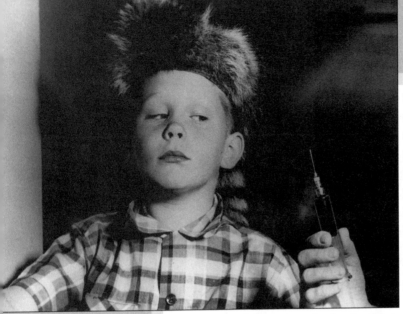

through person-to-person contact; Winkman also observed that those who were paralyzed were only a small percentage of the infected population. In 1908, in Germany, Karl Landsteiner showed that monkeys could be infected with polio even though they were not naturally susceptible, thus providing an animal model that could be used for research. In the United States, Simon Flexner, soon to be director of the Rockefeller Institute for Medical Research, established that seemingly healthy people could be silent carriers of the infection.

While orthopedists and physiatrists studied ways of treating the aftereffects of polio, laboratory researchers tried to devise some means of protecting children from ever catching the disease. The idea was to give a small, controlled exposure to the disease, one that would prompt the body to build its own disease-fighting agents—antibodies. These antibodies in the bloodstream would protect against future encounters with the polio virus.

The principle of immunization had been known for over a century. Like the smallpox vaccine, which grew out of Edward Jenner's first experiments in 1796, a polio vaccine would have to trigger immunity-causing antibodies without creating a severe form of the disease. Researchers would either have to find a weak strain of polio virus that would immunize without paralysis, as cowpox had for smallpox, or they would have to learn how to kill the virus and still have it provoke an immune response, as had been done with influenza, typhoid, and other diseases.

Early experiments led to tragedy. In 1935, before it was known that there were three different types of polio virus or even that the virus circulated in the bloodstream, Dr. John Kolmer designed a vaccine that he believed would give immunity to polio, using a weakened strain of polio virus obtained from the spinal columns of paralyzed monkeys. When the vaccine seemed to work on monkeys, Kolmer injected children, and distributed thousands of doses to other doctors around the country. The results were disastrous. Some children were paralyzed by the injection, and some died. That same year, in separate experiments, Dr. Maurice Brodie developed a vaccine using polio virus killed in Formalin, a chemical solution. Again, early hopes gave way to the realization that the new vaccine, while not as dangerous as Kolmer's, was not effective. Brodie's work had been funded by the proceeds from the first President's Birthday Ball, while Kolmer had been working independently; the National Foundation was blamed for both failures. Kolmer, Brodie, and their colleagues did not realize that there were three separate strains of polio virus. Their techniques had been sloppy, their safety tests inadequate, and their submission to outside evaluation virtually nonexistent. There was still too much they didn't know about polio.

Now the public had two things to fear: polio itself, and false promises of vaccines. In the future, when the National Foundation gave grants to research that might lead to a polio vaccine, it was much more careful about the medical credentials of its advisory board and much more cautious about any work involving human subjects. It was a time to learn about the nature of polio virus, and about all virology. Only then could researchers move ahead toward a vaccine. For the next decade, the National Foundation sponsored research in the fundamentals of virology.

During World War II, as leading research scientists entered the armed forces, Basil O'Connor worried that

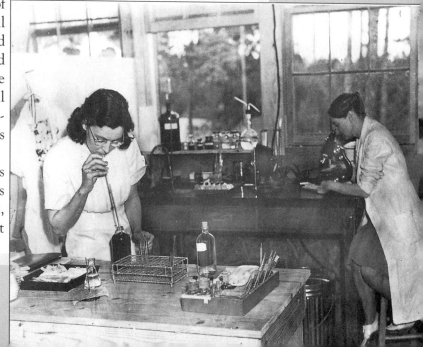

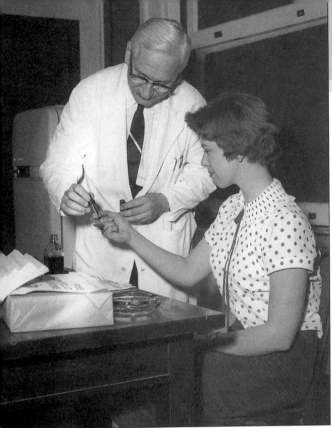

the war effort would halt polio research. Instead, polio became another front within the war. Albert Sabin, already established as a virologist and an authority on polio, joined the Army Medical Corps, assuming his research would be interrupted for the duration of the war. Instead, he found himself assigned to the Mideast, where polio had mysteriously broken out among Allied troops.

Few children in North Africa or around the Mediterranean basin ever seemed to contract infantile paralysis. Working with fellow officer Dr. John Paul, whose laboratory at Yale was devoted to polio virus research, Sabin discovered that polio virus was endemic in the area, but that most children became immune through exposure in infancy when they were still protected by the immunities—the antibodies—they got from their mothers. In the United States and other advanced industrialized areas, modern sanitation had broken the links between children and disease, and many did not come into contact with the crippler until long after infancy, when their mother's protection had worn off and the disease's effects were more severe. U.S. soldiers became sick because they had never had that early, immunizing exposure. At last there was an explanation for the mysterious appearance of polio epidemics at the start of the twentieth century. Unfortunately, it held little comfort for a modern nation desperate to protect its young.

At the same time, progress was finally being made in understanding the disease itself. For decades, scientists had believed a mysterious virus entered the nose and traveled a few inches to the brain, where it attacked the central nervous system. But this was not the case. Studies conducted in the 1940s and 1950s showed that the virus entered the body not through the nose to the brain, but through the mouth into the digestive system. Undetected, the virus moved from the intestines to the blood stream and into the nervous system. There, it attacked the cells that send messages from the brain to the muscles. When the messages stopped, the muscles went dead, and paralysis ensued. The carrier was intestinal waste, feces, and it could spread through the water supply, through unsanitary food handling, and through person-to-person contact.

Meanwhile, new advances in laboratory technology improved the prospects for a polio vaccine. The virus itself could be seen through the new electron microscope, developed in the 1930s and perfected over the next decade. With the centrifuge, the virus could be purified—another crucial step in being able to manufacture a vaccine. But before they could make any vaccine, researchers first had to learn how to produce enough virus to use as their raw material, and how to identify what they had.

All along, vaccine research meant infecting and then dissecting monkey after monkey. Cultivating the virus in live animals was a tedious and frustrating task. The monkey supply was limited and seemed unlikely ever to produce enough usable virus to make a vaccine for mass distribution. A breakthrough came in 1948, in Boston, when John Enders and his colleagues, Thomas Weller and Frederic Robbins, discovered how to grow polio virus in test tubes, using a broth made of monkey kidney. Now, only one monkey was needed to grow hundreds of portions of virus. Next came the need to identify all strains of polio virus, to be sure that any vaccine acted against all of them. Funded by the National Foundation, several laboratories across the country began a three-year program to type all-known samples of polio; at the end, they had confirmed that there were only three strains of the virus.

And every year the epidemics grew larger. Progress came faster, but never fast enough. Eliminating polio had for years been Basil O'Connor's passion. In the summer of 1950 it became his obsession. His daughter Bettyann, a young mother of five, called and said, "Daddy, I've got some of your polio." For the rest of her life, she was confined to a wheelchair. O'Connor had served during World War II as the director of the American Red Cross, but now he was devoting all of his energy to the polio cause. In the past, the search for a polio vaccine had been hampered by ignorance and early mistakes. In the 1950s, the push toward prevention was further complicated by passionate arguments about whether the best vaccine would be made from inactivated, "killed" virus, or from attenuated live virus.

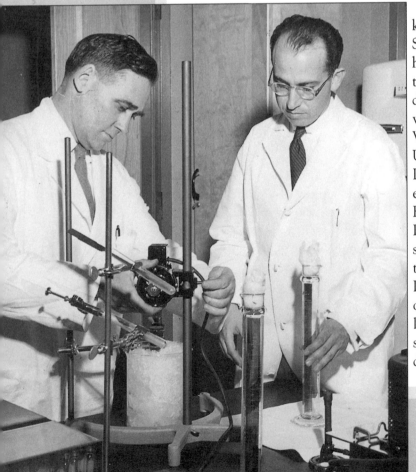

The leading proponent of a killed-virus vaccine was Jonas Salk, a young virologist who had worked on the virus-typing project. Salk had produced "killed virus" influenza vaccines during and after World War II, working at the University of Michigan under Dr. Thomas Francis, a leading epidemiologist and virologist. He came to the University of Pittsburgh and applied these same techniques to polio. At the University of Cincinnati, Dr. Albert Sabin was developing a different vaccine, following methods used against smallpox and rabies: to develop a mild, harmless strain of the virus, and from it make a vaccine that would cause a mild, harmless infection that would then confer lifetime immunity. This method was the one favored by most medical opinion.

Each approach had its advantages. "Killed virus" could be developed faster, and, if done properly, was entirely safe. "Live-virus" vaccine might take longer to perfect, but experience showed that a live-virus vaccine brought lasting immunity. No one was sure how long the immunity from a killed-virus vaccine would last. Some argued that the live-virus vaccine had a substantial public health benefit, since the weakened virus could pass from the vaccinated person to the unvaccinated population; in the same way that a disease could be contagious, so could a protective, mild infection. Opponents countered that a live-virus product might revert to virulence, either in the bloodstream of the vaccinated person or as it passed through the community. If that happened, it might cause the very disease it was supposed to prevent.

Like earlier researchers, Salk and Sabin each were motivated by the sincere belief that his particular method would provide superior immunity—and by an equally natural desire to make sure that his work was not eclipsed by an inferior but earlier announcement by a scientific rival. The medical race to stop the grim rise of polio victims was matched by the personal race to gain the good will, public acceptance, and funding for future research that would come with being first to develop a safe and effective polio vaccine.

As Salk moved rapidly toward his "killed-virus" solution, Albert Sabin grew increasingly agitated. He patronized Salk. And Salk, in turn, could be brash toward Sabin and others in the medical establishment. They weren't in competition—each had his own approach—but their relationship was taking an ever harder edge.

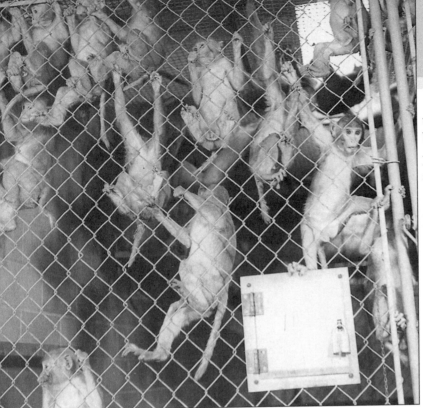

Animal tests showed that Salk's vaccine would build antibodies to the polio virus. But monkeys are ... monkeys. The real test was whether the vaccine would work on humans. Since most adults had acquired immunity at some time, vaccine trials would have to be conducted on children. The mistakes of the 1930s had not been forgotten. No one was going to inoculate children again without being absolutely sure it was safe. Too much caution was equally perilous, though, as any summer headline would reveal. In the days when newspapers reported the daily toll of polio epidemics on the front page, in numbers that seemed to only go up, the campaign against polio gained even more urgency. Haste could be dangerous, but so could delay.

In the early 1950s, at the height of the population explosion known as the baby boom, polio epidemics were rising at an even more explosive rate. In 1933 there had been five thousand new cases of paralytic polio. Ten years later that figure had more than doubled. By 1946, the count was twenty-five thousand new cases. In 1948—twenty-seven thousand. In 1950, it was thirty-three thousand. In 1952, the toll was fifty-nine thousand cases. The shadow of polio was falling across every town in America.

By then, polio epidemics were second only to the atomic bomb in surveys of what Americans feared most. Bomb and virus alike were terrible agents of destruction that might arrive at any moment to devastate a family, a community, or an entire nation. The disease seemed like an omnipresent threat, and its cure became a national responsibility. Epidemics struck other countries, but never as heavily as here. America was the center of polio, and the place where people knew they must work first, and fastest, to end it. And so they did. They gave their time and money to help the growing swell of victims and to find a way to stem the rising tide of injury. When the call came, they even volunteered their children, millions of them, to test a new vaccine. The fear that had once driven Americans apart was now the force that pulled them together.

In the spring of 1952, after two years of preparation, Jonas Salk went to a nearby institution devoted to the rehabilitation of crippled children, and gave the patients his vaccine. Then he checked their blood to see if the injection had increased their antibodies. Almost all of his test subjects had already had polio, though not all had necessarily been exposed to all three strains of the virus. Still, the risks were low, and the possibility of showing that his vaccine could "boost" immunity to even higher levels would be an important first step in human testing. Although sure of his work, Salk nevertheless admitted, "when you inoculate children, you don't sleep well for two or three months."

The most remarkable thing about Salk's early trials in the Pittsburgh area was how few people knew that they were even being held. No one supervised his work, and almost no one even knew what he had done. Then, in January of 1953, Salk traveled to an exclusive polio conference, sponsored by the National Foundation, where he presented a scientific paper entitled, "Studies In Human Subjects On Active Immunization Against Poliomyelitis." The title may have looked routine, but the full import of his work immediately dawned on the

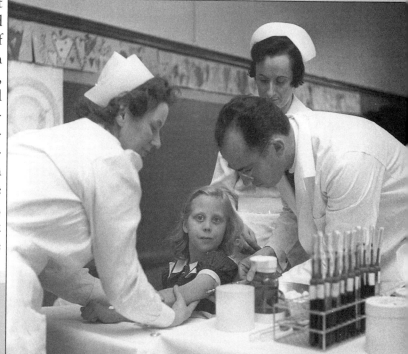

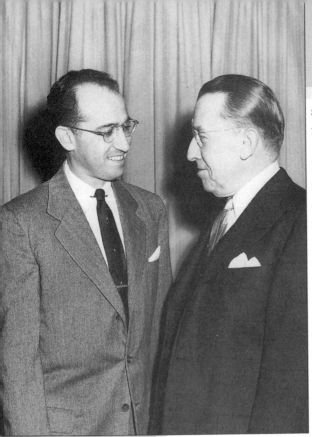

assembled scientists, all of them seasoned polio researchers. Jonas Salk had tested children.

Over the next year, as Salk expanded his local tests to subjects who had not had polio, with entirely safe results, the National Foundation advisors debated moving to the next step—a massive field trial with children from all over the country. The only way to know if his vaccine was effective was to give it to children in an area where an epidemic would occur the following summer, and the only way to be sure that would happen was to vaccinate thousands of children across the country. Sabin protested, insisting any killed-virus vaccine would only provide short-term immunity, thus creating a false sense of security while leaving the population unprotected from future epidemics.

O'Connor hesitated. How could they possibly move forward? Yet, how could they not? And what about all those nagging, "what if's...?" Did Salk really know how long "killed-virus" immunity would last? What if it wore off and left the children who got it at risk all over again? What if his vaccine somehow interfered with the normal immune system, leaving children even more exposed to the disease than before? What if the fluid that held the virus caused allergic reactions or cancer? Finally, O'Connor ended an uneasy silence of indecision. He looked up during one of the many interminable meetings and he spoke of how many thousands of children would be paralyzed by polio every summer they delayed. For his part, O'Connor felt the time had come to move forward to a national field trial.

In a way that is no longer possible, the decision was Basil O'Connor's to make. He needed no government approval to do these tests, though he did seek and finally got a statement of support from the Surgeon General and the Public Health Service. He was paying for the field trial, just as his foundation had paid for the work done by Salk, by Sabin, and by all the advocates and naysayers alike, and he could do as he liked. No matter how uncertain people felt, the National Foundation was supporting a national field trial of Salk's vaccine.

To allay some of the professional fears, that the National Foundation could not successfully run such a complex scientific study, Basil O'Connor enlisted the distinguished epidemiologist Dr. Thomas Francis to be in charge of evaluating whether or not the vaccine worked. Francis imposed his own set of conditions. The first stipulation was that the field trial would have to be a double-blind, placebo-controlled trial, with half the children getting a placebo and half the real vaccine, and neither doctors nor subjects knowing who got what. The second was that all information on the results was to come to Francis' Vaccine Evaluation Center in Ann Arbor, Michigan. The third was that nobody—not Basil O'Connor, Jonas Salk, or Albert Sabin, not the President, Congress, or Centers for Disease Control, not the American Medical Association, or any particular doctor or parent—would have any information until Francis was ready to issue his final report. The field trial would be a huge public event, the largest scientific study ever held, but the evaluation would be very private.

Even with Thomas Francis in charge, opposition to the Salk vaccine trials increased. Sabin went to Congress to testify against it. He wrote to Salk that the "killed-virus" vaccine was "potentially unsafe" and would ruin his career. Others were more alarmist. Walter Winchell used his national radio program to spread the rumor that the National Foundation was stockpiling "little white coffins." For millions of parents, however, the debates over whether one vaccine was superior to another missed the point, which was that salvation was perhaps at hand. To them, the 1954 Salk vaccine field trials were not a risk, but a precious opportunity to have their children protected before

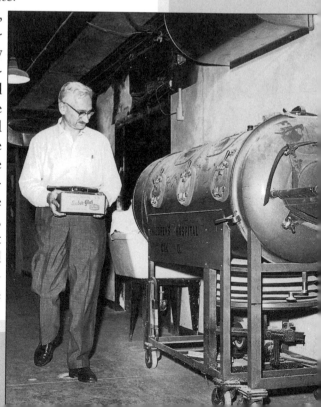

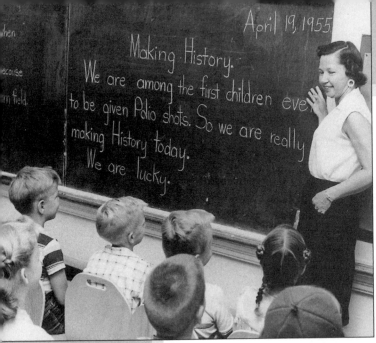

On the chalkboard:
April 19, 1955

Making History.

We are among the first children ever to be given Polio shots. So we are really making History today.

We are lucky.

another epidemic season passed. Many more families volunteered than could take part. They wanted their children to be "Polio Pioneers," blazing a trail through the wilderness of fear.

Salk's killed-virus vaccine was tested on 1.8 million schoolchildren in the spring and summer of 1954. Some received vaccine, some got placebo, and some served as observed controls, children who got no inoculation but whose health was monitored for comparison. Twenty thousand doctors, forty thousand nurses, fifty thousand teachers, and two hundred thousand other volunteers picked up vaccine, delivered children, wiped their tears, and distributed the lollipops and souvenir buttons emblazoned "Polio Pioneer." The field trail of 1954 was unprecedented in its size and its prominence. A Gallup poll showed that nine out of every ten Americans knew about it, more people than knew the full name of the President of the United States.

Even while the field trial was taking place, O'Connor was making plans for the future. If the vaccine worked, there would be a huge demand for more before the polio season of 1955. Afraid that time would be short, the National Foundation borrowed money and ordered $9 million worth of additional vaccine from the companies that had manufactured the field trial supplies.

Months would pass before O'Connor knew if the investment had any value. Records of polio cases during the summer of 1954 had to be amassed from across the country, and then compared with the coded records of which children had in fact received vaccine. Hundreds of thousands of punch cards and endless statistical tables had to be compiled. Then, at 10:00 A.M. on April 12, 1955, the tenth anniversary of the death of President Roosevelt, Thomas Francis announced to a throng of dignitaries and an even larger mass of reporters that the Salk vaccine was safe and effective. By 5:30 that afternoon, the federal government issued the license for commercial manufacture.

Americans wanted a hero and they had one in Jonas Salk. Young and soft-spoken, he seemed the model of the scientific savior. He was featured on television and radio programs and on the front page of newspapers around the world. He was called to the White House to receive a medal. When asked who owned the vaccine, Salk said modestly, "I'd say it belongs to everyone. I mean, could you patent the sun?"

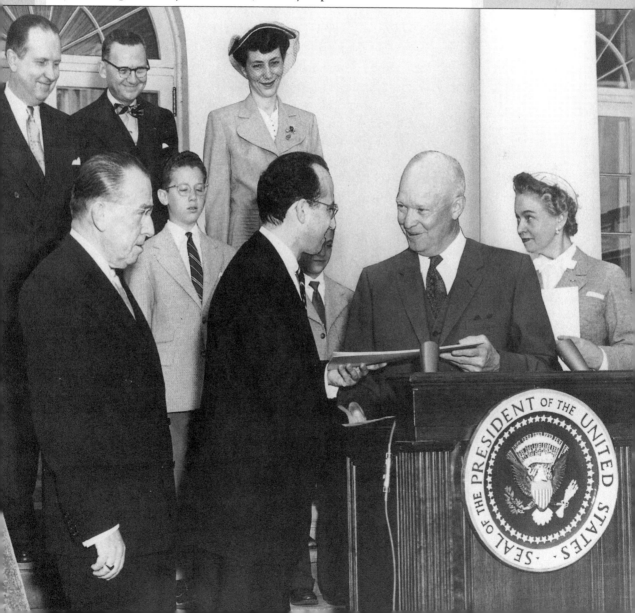

Then, two weeks into nationwide vaccination, some children who had received the Salk shots came down with polio. All vaccinations had to be halted until the source of the problem was found. Working with speed born of despair, health officials soon discovered that nine lots of the killed-virus vaccine produced at the Cutter Laboratories in California were contaminated with live polio virus. Two hundred and four vaccinated children, their siblings, and their playmates had contracted the disease. Fifty children lay paralyzed. Eleven were dead.

After supplies from other manufacturers were found to be safe, nationwide vaccination did resume, but the Cutter incident, as it was called, destroyed the elation felt only two weeks before. Jonas Salk was devastated by the knowledge that children had been injured by his vaccine, and dismayed that the episode had also destroyed the momentum of the vaccination program. Within two years of the introduction of the killed-virus vaccine, polio incidence dropped by 80 percent in areas where everyone was vaccinated, but some people weren't getting their shots.

In part, it was fear of more problems with the contaminated vaccine. More often, failure to be vaccinated came from a strange but widespread form of psychological immunity, where the sheer existence of a vaccine seemed to remove the threat of disease. People felt safe again, even though they were not. Huge public campaigns had to be launched to get people to take the life-saving medicine they had so eagerly awaited.

Perhaps the problem was the vaccination format, which called for three separate injections. Perhaps a simpler type of vaccine could be used. By 1959, Albert Sabin was ready to test his "live-virus" vaccine, which was taken orally. To have meaningful results he needed a population that had never been vaccinated, living in a place known to have polio.

He went to Russia, the country he had left as a young child when his family emigrated to America. There had been epidemics of polio in Russia since the start of the century. Even in the depths of the Cold War, Soviet doctors invited Sabin to set up a huge program of giving his oral vaccine. Sabin knew that if this program succeeded, the U.S.

Public Health Service would have to take note and consider "live-virus" vaccine for distribution in America.

In the next two years, seventy-seven million Russians took the "live-virus" vaccine. Although some questioned the accuracy of the Russian data, the test was judged a success by world health experts. In 1961, the American Medical Association endorsed Sabin's oral polio vaccine for use in the United States.

Vaccination clinics were set up in schools and churches, and even in shopping center parking lots. Entire communities were urged to come out on a single day to get their vaccine, usually administered in a single gulp of sweet liquid or on a vaccine-saturated sugar cube. Within five years, the oral vaccine had replaced the Salk injected vaccine as the preference of doctors and public health officials.

To their lifelong mutual chagrin, Salk's name was forever associated with the polio vaccine, but Sabin's was the formula that was used. In recent years, the World Health Organization has started to recommend that children be vaccinated with both—first a killed-virus vaccine to create immunity, and then a live-virus one for guaranteed long-term protection. In the clash of personalities between Salk and Sabin, and amidst the swirling claims and counterclaims for each vaccine, it is important to remember that both work very well. In the forty years since the last polio epidemics, polio incidence in America has fallen from thousands of cases a year to less than ten. This is truly an extraordinary triumph.

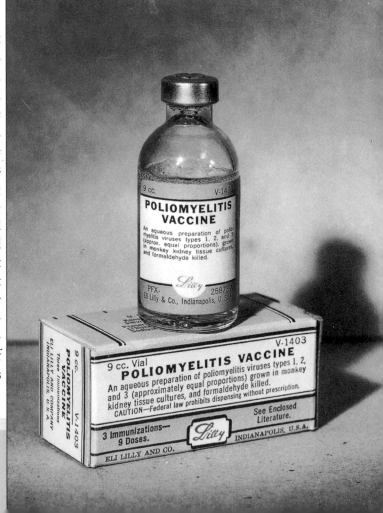

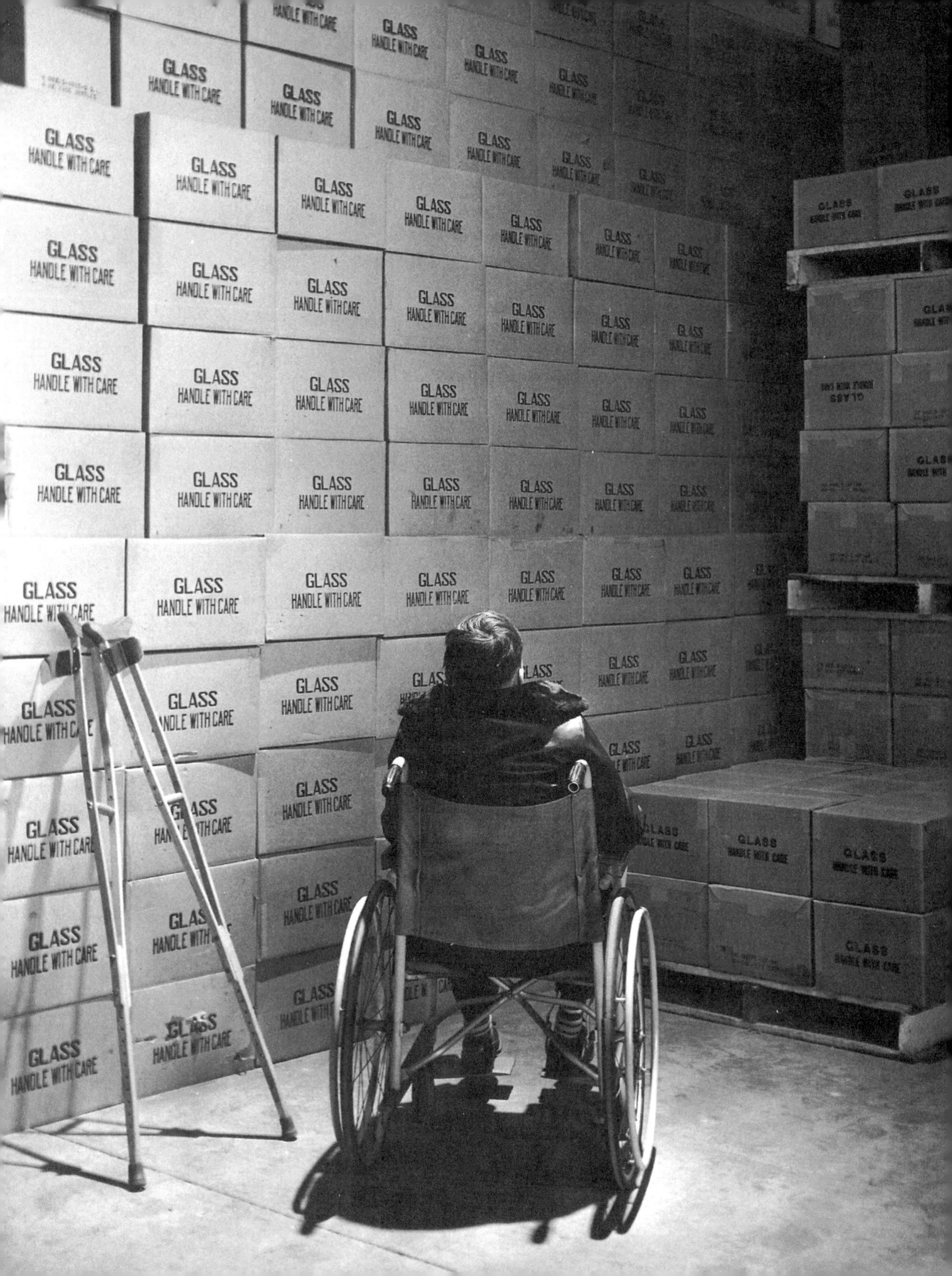
GLASS
HANDLE WITH CARE

Voices
John Troan

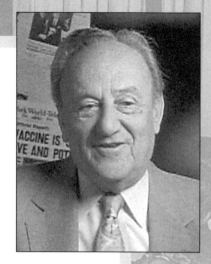

John Troan was a medical reporter and science reporter for the *Pittsburgh Press*. He covered the development of the Salk vaccine from its earliest beginnings through to the 1955 announcement of its success.

Tell me about the first time you met Jonas Salk.

I had just been assigned to the University of Pittsburgh Medical Center by the *Pittsburgh Press*. Nobody had paid attention to the medical center before that, so I was always hunting stories. An assistant dean was one of my great feeders of information, and this particular Friday afternoon he said, 'Why don't you go see Jonas Salk?' And I said, 'Who the heck is Jonas Salk?' He says, 'He's a young firebrand that the dean has brought in from the University of Michigan to set up a virus research lab. Just go there, and tell him I sent you.' So I went and sat down with Jonas. He was working on an influenza vaccine. He was trying to extend the efficacy of the vaccine by adding mineral oil to it, and he was about to test it on something like twelve thousand soldiers at Fort Dix, New Jersey. So we talked about it and he says 'Now, do you mind if I read your story before it's printed?' And I said, 'Well, to tell you the truth I'm so new at this game that I do ask the doctor or scientist to look over the material for factual accuracy. But you just told me you're leaving tonight for Fort Dix. I'm writing the story for the Sunday paper.' I said, 'Listen, if I foul up the story, don't speak to me again.' Well, I didn't know he was going to hit the jackpot. I would never have made that offer. But I did write the story. And he was so intent on checking it that he must have been walking the boardwalk in Atlantic City that Sunday afternoon, picked up the *Pittsburgh Press*, and read the story. I got a telegram, 'Splendid job, thanks.' I still have the telegram.

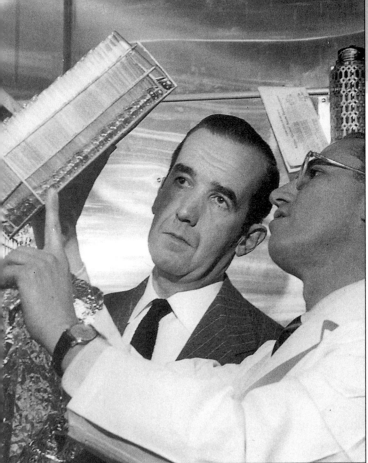

He was uncomfortable with news people. He was so intent on doing his work that he didn't want to waste time speaking to anybody in the news media. And he was concerned that they would publish inaccurately or prematurely, as he would put it. I don't know why we hit it off so well except for that first story, where he began to trust me. And so we would meet. I would go to the Bamboo Garden in Pittsburgh. I learned to eat Chinese food for lunch because that's what Jonas liked. And I'd pretend I just bumped into him accidentally, although one of his colleagues told me where I could find him. So I would sit there in the booth talking to him about how things were going.

How did Salk get into the hunt for a polio vaccine?

He came to Pittsburgh about 1947, and he was given a blank check to set up a lab and do whatever he wanted. He worked on the flu vaccine for that first year. And then the polio foundation came in and signed him up, plus people at Kansas and Utah and Southern California, to find out exactly how many types of polio virus there were. It took three years to determine that there were just three types of virus. By the middle of 1952, just about eighteen months later, he was already testing the vaccine on the children at D. T. Watson's home. As you can tell from the timetable, he immediately jumped. He wasn't going to wait for anybody else.

Where was Salk in the world of polio scientists?

Salk was concerned because back in the 1930s someone developed a polio vaccine that crippled about a dozen children. So Salk went against conventional wisdom when he decided that he would develop a dead virus instead of a live-virus vaccine. But essentially he was doing this to be safe. He thought that would be the safest way to proceed. And that was his first concern. He first tried it on animals, then he tried it on humans who had already partial immunity to polio because they had been crippled by it, then he went on to test it on people who had no immunity at all. And there were many who said it would never work. As a matter of fact the National Academy of Sciences never accepted him for membership, which is a scientific tragedy.

Talk about the private side of Salk during this time, and how he dealt with the public interest in his work.

Jonas Salk was always an intense person. He was a man possessed once he could see the prize out there. And he just worked night and day. He didn't like to fly at that time, and he would take a train overnight from Pittsburgh to New York. He'd work in New York, then he'd come back and I'd call his home. He had given me his private phone number. And his wife would answer and say, 'You don't know Jonas, he went right to the lab.' And so he would be spending night and day there trying to get things going. He said to me at one time, 'God, they're just pushing hard.' I said, 'What do you mean, "they"?' And he said, 'I think Basil O'Connor wants to be sure that this is solved while he's still alive.' He said, 'I don't want to be rushed into anything. I want to take this step by step, just the way it should be done.' And he said, 'Safety is first.'

Once the word was getting around that he had a vaccine to work with, *Life* magazine wanted to come in and take pictures of Dr. Salk in the lab. This had to be in 1952. And he said no. Now, the *Life* stringer in Pittsburgh was my assistant city editor. So he came to me and asked if I could help. So I called Salk and said, 'I'm just calling you because my boss asked me to.' He said, 'I don't like to give up all this time.' I said, 'It's only going to take from ten 'til noon.' So he agreed. The *Life* magazine photographer was accompanied by a photographer from the National Foundation who was taking pictures as a backup. So they're telling him to raise his vials of virus. 'Little higher, doctor, little higher.' He banged them against the metal overhead. The flask broke and the virus spilled on the floor. We broke the 100-yard dash getting out of there. We came back and Salk was mopping the floor, and he was laughing. When they finally left at three, he said to me, 'Two hours, huh? I'm glad this is a leap year, I can make up the lost day.' The addendum is that the next day a researcher from *Life* magazine called and said, 'I hate to ask this, but could you ask Salk's lab to check and see whether there's a bag of film left there?' I said, 'Oh, my God.' *Life* magazine wound up using the foundation film. Never found the other film.

How did Salk begin testing his vaccine?

He wanted to first take people who already had some immunity so the risk was lower. If you were already immune to one type of polio, if the vaccine went bad, there were only two chances out of three that it would go, and not three out of three, that it would harm someone. And so they went to the D. T. Watson home for children. Also Salk had a working relationship with Dr. Jesse Wright, who sold the whole project to the director of the home. And they signed up all forty children who were there, recovering from their bouts with polio, and lined them up one day. There were three young children at the head of the line. The children were crying, and so a young man named Bill Kirkpatrick stepped in front to show them it wouldn't hurt. He got the first needle. And that's how he became my hero, number one polio volunteer. Bill went on to become an Episcopal priest.

Then Salk went to the Polk home, where there were children who had not been out in society and the suspicion was they had no immunity. And that was true. They had zero immunity to polio. That would show that the vaccine was not just a booster to your natural immunity, but would give you initial immunity and would work in anybody. And he got great results there.

After he was sure it was safe, he gave himself the vaccine, he gave his wife the vaccine, and he gave his three sons the vaccine. And the sons didn't like it. They cried. I talked to his wife and she said, 'Oh, he doesn't give them whooping cough shots. We go to a pediatrician for all the shots. But Jonas did these.' And so Darrell and Jonathan and Peter all got the Salk shots from daddy.

Salk, Sabin, and the Search for a Vaccine

182

Salk told me later that after the initial test he was very distressed for two or three weeks because he wanted to be sure nothing went wrong with them. He said, 'When you give some of the polio vaccine for the first time, you just...you're on pins and needles waiting for the results.' And after three weeks everything just turned fine. All the immunity levels went up, nobody got paralyzed. He was on his way.

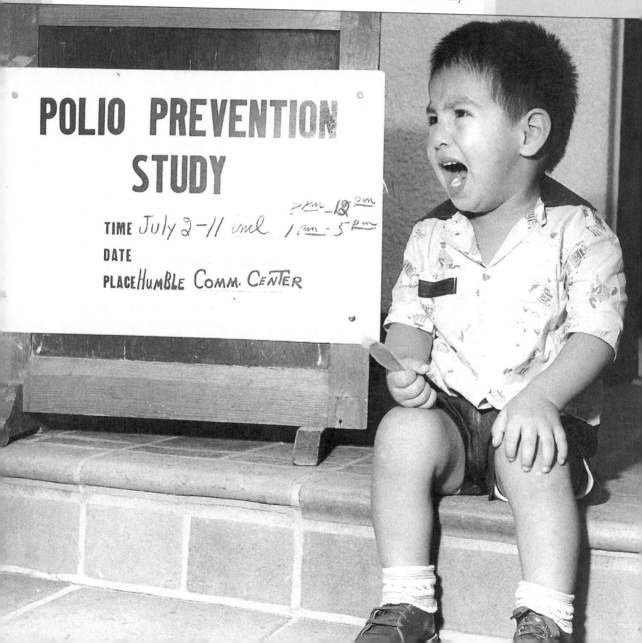

POLIO PREVENTION STUDY

TIME July 2–11 incl.   2pm–12pm   1pm–5pm
DATE
PLACE Humble Comm. Center

But he was getting pressure from the foundation.

He was getting pressure from everyone. I mean, people were anxious. 'Let's get going' and 'Do we really have the answer?' And 'Let's stop the epidemics.' Because every summer, as soon as the first polio case was reported, the fear would build and escalate immediately. Imagine having children in your household and one comes home with a crick in the neck. And the first thing you think is, 'It's got to be polio.' And it takes time to determine whether it is polio. And by that time they tell you, 'No, it's not polio' you feel like you've already gone through it. Just the realization that this could happen to you, there was no prevention. So once it was announced that Salk had something working, why, everybody was grasping for it.

When did the results of his research start coming out?

I didn't know the details, all I kept hearing was, 'Things are going well' from Jim Lewis [who worked with Salk]. 'But keep the lid on.' So I played the game, I kept the lid on, and just waited. There was really nothing concrete that I could write about. I was hinting in stories that things were working but never said, 'Yes, we already have a vaccine going.' And finally in January of 1953 all kinds of rumors were going on. So I happened to go to New York to the National Foundation and that's when the story broke. In fact, that night Dr. Weaver, from the National Foundation, announced to the Board of Directors that they have one. And I believe the following night Jonas Salk went on the air to speak for himself. He had already filed the actual scientific report with the *Journal of the American Medical Association*. And that's how the rumors start. Editors read it and they start talking.

Tell me about 'The Scientist Speaks for Himself.'

He wanted that opportunity to speak for himself. Now, Jonas spoke in question marks a lot of times. Instead of actual concrete statements he would ask questions as he was doing something. So he didn't come across too clearly. But I think a lot of the science writers were able to translate what he was saying into understandable English. I know sometimes he would answer a question and one of the reporters said to him, 'Gee, Jonas, you really ran around the mulberry bush on that one.' He said, 'You guys taught me to do that.'

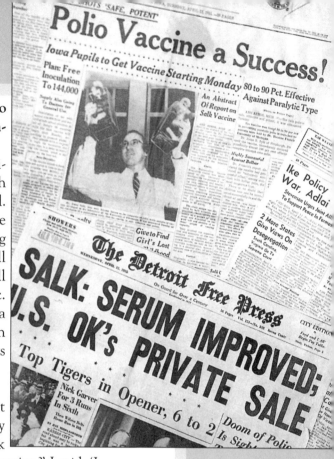

Do you think speaking on the radio separated him from the scientific community?

I think there was resentment that a scientist would come out with a public speech rather than filing a report first in a journal. And this was almost simultaneous. Because he spoke one night and the next morning the *AMA Journal* was out. There's still some of that in scientific circles. They still don't want people talking to the public. They want the researchers to report in a journal, a technical journal where they can read all the technical ifs, ands, and buts and pick it apart, challenge it.

Then the pressure was really on.

Then it began. They began calling it the Salk vaccine. And he was distressed by that. He said, 'Why did you call it the Salk vaccine? Why don't you call it the Pitt vaccine?' I said, 'Jonas, everybody's now calling it the Salk vaccine, it's a beautiful little word—it fits in a headline.' He said, 'Well Pitt is even shorter than Salk.' I tried 'Pitt vaccine' several times, and it just didn't take. Not with the foundation and not with anyone else.

Let's talk about Dr. Sabin.

Dr. Sabin was insistent that a dead virus would not work, and that a live-virus vaccine would produce better immunity and work longer than dead-virus vaccines. There were people who pointed out that the yellow fever vaccine was a live-virus. It works about the best of live-virus vaccines. [Sabin] was also upset that the foundation was putting more of its money on the Salk vaccine than on the Sabin vaccine. And I recall walking down the boardwalk in Atlantic City at a medical meeting one year, and he was walking ahead of me with Roland Berg, who at the time was the director of public relations for the foundation and later became the medicine editor for *Look* magazine. So he was waving his arms and gesticulating, and when it was all over I said to Roland, 'What's with Al Sabin today?' He said, 'He was telling me that he would've had the vaccine first if Basil O'Connor had not given support to Salk ahead of Sabin.' I think O'Connor did it because he was worried about safety and he thought, 'If you can do it with a dead virus, why bet on the live virus?'

Sabin mounted his own campaign.

Well, Sabin criticized the fact that the first group of children who had been tested [with the Salk vaccine] had partial immunity. Sabin spoke at a medical meeting and said that all Salk had proved was that his vaccine was a good booster, that it didn't prove that it gave initial immunity. And I remember calling Salk on the phone for his reaction to that and he said, 'That bastard.' And he said, 'He's reacting to the published report. I filled him in on triple zeros—children who had no immunity at all, and how the vaccine worked well in them. And he's ignoring that so that he can criticize it as just a booster shot.' But eventually, in their later years they talked to each other.

Sabin had opposed field trials?

I don't recall how actively he opposed them but he certainly was unhappy that they were going ahead with them. He said it wasn't ready, and even if it were it wouldn't prove much, because he still thought the immunity would not be long-lasting.

Back to Salk: How did he do the field trials?

Well, before the national field trials he was urged to do some preliminary testing in the Pittsburgh area, which he did. He got all these children at schools in the area and personally began giving the inoculations himself. And that was about 5,000. This was primarily not for safety—he was already sure of the safety—this was for potency. There were different products coming from different drug houses, and he was trying to determine which ones would work best in the national field trials. Unfortunately, there was not enough of the top-notch vaccine for the field trials. Some of the batches were weaker than others. But they all produced immunity and they all proved to be safe. And I think they had about 1.8 million children all together. About 450,000 got the actual vaccine, and another 450,000 got dummy shots. These were

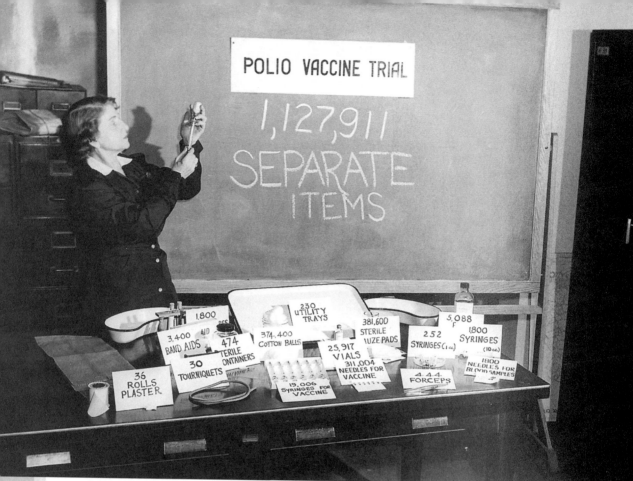

all checked secretly, even the families didn't know whether the children got the real vaccine or not.

It was a magnificent, cooperative effort, with all these health directors throughout the country getting all these children and the school people selling it to the parents, telling them, 'Go ahead and do that.' Of course, the fear of polio was so great that the likelihood that you're going to finally put an end to this disease drove a lot of parents to say, 'Yes, hurry up! Do it!' I don't think they ran into any difficulty getting volunteers. But then, before the field trials started, one Sunday night Walter Winchell came out with a scary report and said, 'Listen to this! Children are about to start getting this vaccine which can be a killer!' I remember talking to Salk the next day, and he was upset, of course. He said something like, 'Winchell should stick to propaganda or rumors and not dabble in medicine.'

Aside from Winchell's 'little white coffins' broadcast, what were the challenges of a field trial of that size?

The problem was organizing. We didn't have computers then, and it did take almost the whole year to finally get the results. But they did everything before June because they were afraid that the regular polio season would then interfere with the results: you wouldn't know whether the child got polio because of the vaccine or in spite of it. So they stopped them, and then at the end of October they began compiling the results.

By February, everybody was trying to guess whether the vaccine worked. But it was obvious that it was working, because if it hadn't been working we would have heard stories about children being crippled all over the place. We all thought 'It's working.' The PR men in the drug houses were saying, 'Everything's cooking well' or something

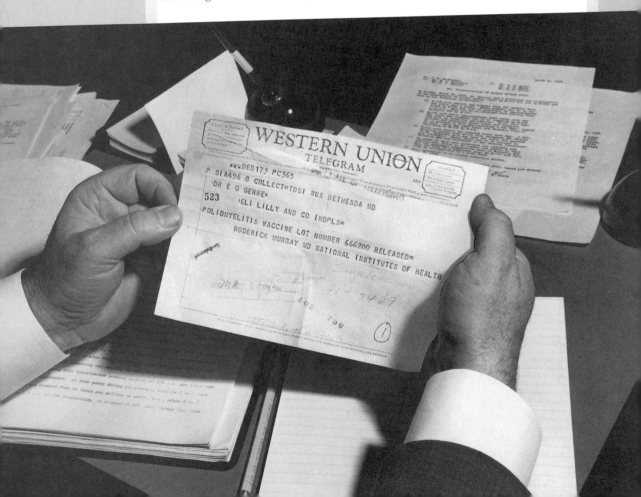

like that. We had no idea how well. In April, I got a call from Dr. Lewis in Salk's lab, and he said, 'John, Dr. Workman's here.' I said, 'Who's Dr. Workman?' He said, 'He's the head of the division of biologic standards at the National Institutes of Health and they license vaccines. He's in the room with Jonas and they're going over the protocols.' So I said, 'Wow,' and began calling all the drug companies and put together a story saying that this is it, it'll be licensed within ten days. It isn't perfect—nothing is perfect—but it's good enough to be licensed. And that was about April 4.

This was immediately followed by the announcement in Ann Arbor.

We all went to Ann Arbor. We were in this big hall, about five hundred scientists and health directors invited to attend. It must have been five hundred news people or maybe a thousand, all over the place. And they brought the report in on dollies, and newsmen were jumping over each other and screaming, 'It works! It works! It works!' The whole place was bedlam. And this is where I saw one of the doctors with tears in his eyes, he was so emotionally moved. I happened to sit next to a fellow who was chain smoking—Edward R. Murrow. He was going to have Jonas on camera that night, and he was working hard, trying to figure out what questions to ask him. 'What now, Dr. Salk?' But it was sheer bedlam, and some of the scientists who were there said, 'This is no way to announce anything.'

What happens to Jonas Salk after the announcement?

Well he's beset by everybody. I think he tried to get away for three days or so, some place where nobody would find him. Meanwhile the University of Pittsburgh is being overwhelmed. The White House wants him, everybody wants him. Ed Murrow had had him the night of the announcement, and so now everybody wants a piece of Jonas Salk. Congress wants to give him a medal, and the state legislature wants to give him a Salk grant, a chair, to head up the Department of Preventive Medicine at the University of Pittsburgh. And he lost his voice from talking so much. He said to me, 'Why are they after me?' I think when Jonas Salk developed the vaccine, I believe his salary was $9,500. And I said to him 'Jonas, why are you in research? You could be in private practice making a lot more than that.' And he said to me, 'Why did Mozart write music?' And he said, 'This is my hobby, and I'm glad to be paid for it.' But then he said, 'Why do they want to give me more money to be the head of a department, to be an administrator, when I don't know whether I can administer, and I don't think I'd like it. Why don't they just give the money to do what I proved I could do and want to keep doing?' Then he left and set up the institute in La Jolla.

Salk was never accepted in the scientific community.

Well, he never played politics. I'm not sure that he was ever a member of the American Medical Association. He just stuck to his own marbles there and never bothered trying to make the kind of friends that you need to politic.

Do you think he suffered from that?

I don't know that he suffered. I think he's more famous than any of the others, and I don't think the public cares whether you're a member of the National Academy of Sciences or not. I think the Nobel Prize rightfully went to Enders, who paved the way for many vaccines, not just the polio vaccine. But I think prizes have gone to other people for lesser accomplishments than Salk. I mean, if you look back, over the forty years the polio vaccine and the ones that followed have saved about 70,000 people from being killed, close to a million from being paralyzed. And millions and millions of Americans from being emotionally paralyzed every summer. And this is for about $25 million from the National Foundation. I think it's the most cost effective investment in medical research in American history.

Don Wegemer

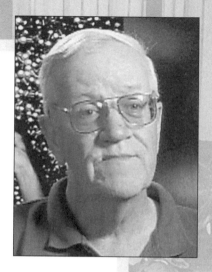

Don Wegemer was one of Jonas Salk's laboratory assistants from the early days at the University of Pittsburgh. Before the vaccine was tested on humans, Dr. Salk inoculated all of his assistants, including Wegemer, with the yet-to-be-proven killed-virus vaccine.

Tell me about Dr. Salk's background with the polio virus.

Well, Salk had typed influenza viruses with Tommy Francis before this even started. He did an excellent job influenza typing. He made a good flu vaccine even before the polio vaccine. And the University of Pittsburgh said, 'Hey let's bring this guy in, he's good. We want to set up something that we can work on viruses.'

Describe the laboratory.

Our laboratory was on the first and the basement floors in the municipal hospital, which was the communicable disease hospital for Allegheny County, primarily for Pittsburgh. The floors above us were people with infectious diseases. On the fourth and fifth floors there were people that had the effects of polio. There were people in iron lungs in rooms with wheelchairs, braces, canes, and things for mobility. Our laboratory was set up inside a conference room on the first floor. It was divided into six small laboratories, with a hallway, and at the end of the hallway there was a supply room. Dr. Salk's office was about two doors down from the main entrance near the elevator shaft. The other part of our laboratory was in the basement, which actually was the morgue area for the hospital. So we used to store some of our equipment in the slide-out drawers where they used to store bodies overnight. Of course, people weren't there at that time. That lab was primarily our kitchen area, and the area in which the monkey kidney

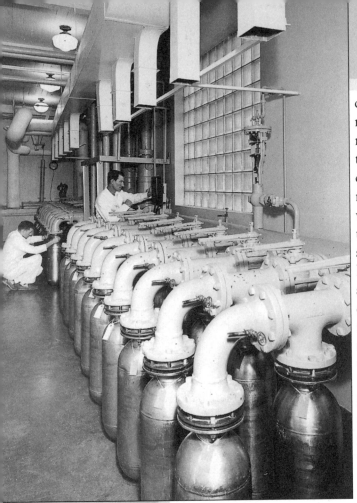

cells were prepared. We had three rooms down there, and in one of the rooms was our incubators. The incubators were essentially handmade, because at that time we didn't have the massive equipment or techniques that we have now. So actually our incubators were old egg incubators. They had stainless steel shelves, which held these large toxin bottles. [They were constructed] to keep things moving in a circular motion. The idea for the motion was that you had maximum chance of contact between cell and virus.

What was it like working in the lab, knowing that at the same time there were children in hospitals, in iron lungs, children dying while you were working on a vaccine.

It was quite an incentive. When you work in the medical field you see people that need help and you say, 'Boy, there's something I can do to help 'em, let's do it.' And this was the idea, we've got all these people above us in the hospital, we've got friends, relatives, childhood playmates. I had a great friend, for example, who was paralyzed by polio, poor guy. So let's do something down here to help them. At the time there were many people working on the viruses, trying to isolate different viruses. Salk said, 'Okay, we've got the people here who can do the job that we have in mind to do. Let's go do it.' If you need inspiration you don't have to look to heaven, you can just look above to the floors above you and see these people that need help. And we've got the facilities to do it now, we know what we're doing. We can alleviate a lot of this suffering. Fifty thousand people or so a year are coming down with polio. Parents are scared to death to put their kids out in the swimming pools, you're in this grip of terror. And how are you going to alleviate it? You're going to make sure that the people that are susceptible to the disease process have protection. And this can be done only with antibodies, which are going to kill the virus.

Monkeys were key to your work. Where were they housed?

We had a monkey colony on the second floor. We'd have anywhere from 100 to 150 monkeys held there, and we had eight chimpanzees. All the monkeys were under quarantine. They were fed their own special diet. We made the monkey food right there in our own laboratory for them so it was prepared with all the vitamins and minerals that were needed. When they were isolated long enough to make sure they didn't have any disease they were separated into individual cages.

What did you do with the monkeys?

The monkeys were used as test animals and also as sources for kidneys. The only cells we could use at that time were primary monkey kidney cells. We couldn't use brains or muscle fiber or any other nerve cell. The monkeys were used to check the virus and make sure it was dead and also to check the efficiency of the virus and activation. This means that we had a virus preparation that we had inactivated with formaldehyde. We think it's dead, but we want to make sure it's dead. So we would inoculate it into a susceptible animal—an animal that's going to come down with all the symptoms of infantile paralysis. So the head of the monkey would be taken, the skin would be pulled back and we would drill into the skull. An injection would be made of the virus preparation. Then the monkey would be put back into its cage and you look for paralysis and death of the monkey. If the virus had been killed by the formal inactivation, the monkey would be perfectly all right.

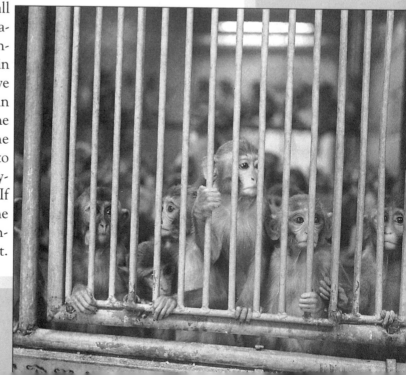

And even if the animal survived it was autopsied and all the organs were looked at to make sure that there was no virus within any of the cells of the monkey's tissue. We used the monkeys up until about 1955.

Tell me about Dr. Salk and his routine with these experiments.

Dr. Salk would walk around and see everybody in the lab. He used to smoke cigarettes like a fiend, and he'd borrow cigarettes from everybody. So everybody would make sure they had packs of cigarettes for him to go into. But he would come into the lab, watch you, and see what's going on. And sometimes it would become annoying, you know, because someone's watching you. So occasionally you just say, 'Dr. Salk, if I'm going to get anything done you're going to have let me go ahead and do what we're doing and then we'll find out.' He was always interested in what everybody was doing and good communication between people. The people would meet with him and we'd have ideas. His main function was to make sure that everybody was doing

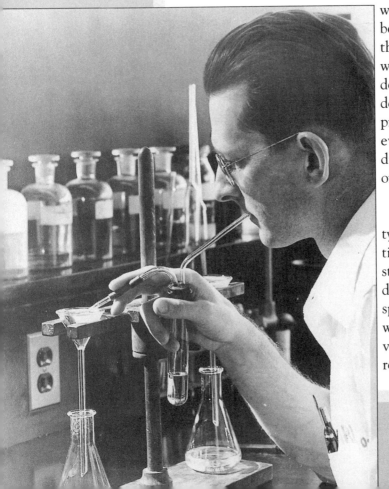

what they said they were doing because in any laboratory you get these rugged individualists who want to go off on tangents. They deviate and do what they want to do, but it isn't helping the overall program. So Salk made sure that everybody was focused and directed. We had a limited amount of time.

Talk about typing the viruses.

There were a number of labs typing the viruses because at this time they didn't know how many strains of viruses there were. And different laboratories got these specimens and they would see what type they were. All of the viruses which were isolated would react either with the type 1 antiserum, type 2, or type 3. There are just three types of polio, which is a good thing to know because if you are immunized with these three strains and there was a wild type out there you'd have no protection. And once you get enough of them together you know that they're going to act the same way.

After identifying three types what happens next?

Salk says we've got these three types of viruses—what are we going to do with them? Why don't we make a vaccine that we can inject into animals, first, to see what's going on and then put them in people and see if we get any responses to it. This is where the pace quickened because all this money was coming in and what was being shown for it? Over this period of time, up into the 1940s you see pictures of wheelchairs and braces and iron lungs, physical therapy and hydro therapy. All of a sudden now we get a break. We now have a virus, we know what's causing it, and the main thing is to stop it from happening rather than to try to cure it. So Salk said, 'Okay, there are other vaccines, we'll follow some of the same things.' Particularly a killed-virus vaccine. So we made the three strains, we inactivated each one separately, then made combinations. [This was] injected into monkeys. The monkeys developed antibodies against the killed-virus vaccine. So we have a vaccine against polio, which, when injected into monkeys, produces antibodies to neutralize the virus. If it works in monkeys, which are primates, it will work in higher primates. This was put into people who already had polio and had survived it and were okay. So they have antibodies against polio and now they are responding to a killed virus by producing more specific antibodies against that particular virus. We tried this often, though a number of people who had not had the disease [also] produced antibodies, and these people weren't getting sick. So the injection of the killed-virus vaccine has induced the people to produce specific antibodies against the dead virus and the same antibodies that work against the dead virus also work against the live virus. So you have people now who have been treated with a vaccine that carries antibodies that are able to inactivate live virus—either type 1, 2, or 3—when they come in contact with it.

Tell me about the field trials.

The vaccine had been made, mostly by us but also by a number of pharmaceutical houses. The field trials involved [about] 1.4 million people. Some of them got non-vaccine and some of them got vaccine, so that when they were tested and examined we could differentiate. Is this thing really working or isn't this working? Because those that aren't getting the vaccine will get the disease, or a certain percentage of them will, but most of them will not get the disease. I was the one who made all of the materials that were used in the field trial testings. The tissue culture medium, the serum, and the reagents were shipped every Monday to twenty different laboratories. We were the only ones at that time who had the ability to make large volumes of tissue culture medium. We had bulk production of tissue culture medium, and ours was the most uniformly controlled. The animal serum that was used in the tissue culture medium was produced on our own farms. We had our own horse and our own cows out there that were the source of the serum. So we would bleed our own animals, which we knew were good for test purposes, and ship these off to people so that there would be no screw-up.

Did Dr. Salk inoculate everyone in the lab?

In 1953, all of the people in the laboratory got the injection of the killed-virus vaccine. Everyone was first bled, their serum antibodies were checked to find out if they had antibodies to it. The general population has antibodies against one or two or even all three types of polio. Then we were given an injection of the virus, re-checked again, and now we have antibodies against all three types.

What was the feeling inside lab during the field trials?

We were all on pins and needles. We wanted to find out what was going on and to make sure that nobody was going to be killed with the stuff that we had provided. The lab was functioning during field trials. We were back in Pittsburgh and the other laboratories were testing the samples. We didn't even see the samples they were testing, but we knew that they were getting them and that we were sending them materials to test their samples. And of course, the results there were going to Tommy Francis at the University of Michigan.

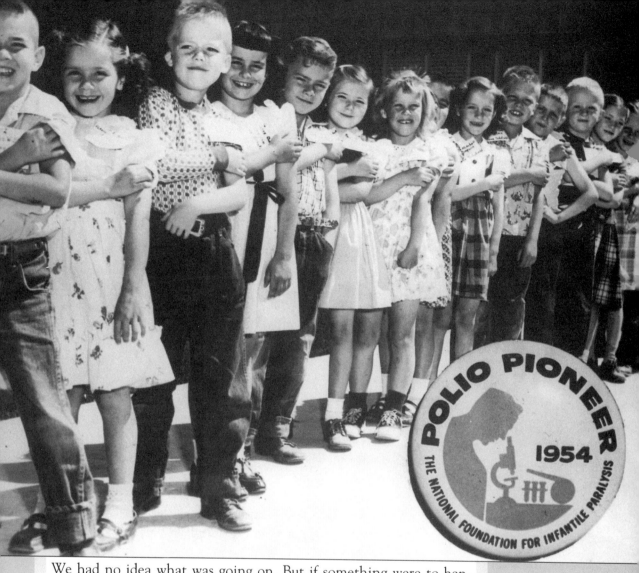

We had no idea what was going on. But if something were to happen, I'm sure we would have known about it.

At what point did Salk think the vaccine was going to work?

About Labor Day, about two years before the field trials started. In 1952 or 1953 at the Watson home, we had some prisoners that were injected with the material in addition to those people at the Watson Home. Prisoners are good subjects—they've got nothing to lose. It was after we had had ours, and after Dr. Salk's own family had had it. So we felt pretty good about it. The anticipation around the field trials was, 'It's going to work.' Other killed vaccines have worked. So we waited for the report to come from Tommy Francis. We knew that it was going to be good, it had to be good because there was nothing we could have done wrong.

No one knew until the day of the announcement what the results would be?

We had no idea, and Salk and Donna and the boys went there, and certain people from the lab went there too. I was back in the lab when I heard it, that the vaccine was 90 percent effective. We were really elated. . . . It's a feeling of, 'Hey! Here's things that have been running rampant for centuries. We now have a mechanism to make sure that it's not going to cause any more problems.' It's a great feeling.

What was the cause of the Cutter incident?

We had these cases of people getting the vaccine coming down with paralytic polio, and the incidence was too high. So we got some of Cutter's vaccine samples and we found out what we thought may be the problem. When you get into finances, people try to make short-cuts—I got it, I'm going to make more of it, and I'm going to make more money. And this was what was happening. 'We got it, we're going to do it our way.' It's very easy to have things nice and controlled when you're doing small amounts of materials. But when you start expanding from small volumes to big volumes and you don't adhere to specifications, you're getting problems.

What was Dr. Salk's reaction to the Cutter incident?

He said something is happening: the specifications have not been done. Something is wrong. He said, 'This is dreadful. I feel terrible. People are trusting me and all of a sudden this is happening to them.' Dr. Salk was very, very dejected. And then we found out what was going on, and the problem was rectified. No problems after that.

Donna Salk

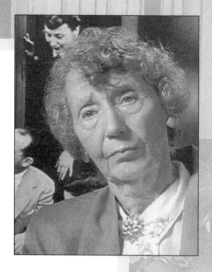

Donna Salk was the wife of Dr. Jonas Salk at the time of the research and discovery of the killed virus polio vaccine. She is the mother of their three sons, Peter, Darrell, and Jonathan, and is accomplished in the field of social work.

Could you talk about what drove Jonas Salk?

Jonas had the idea, from a time when he was quite young, that he wanted to do something that would make a difference to humanity. And so he was fueled by an idealism that was sincere, backed by all the scientific knowledge, and his personality, and his ability to follow through. It was extremely important to him to achieve and that's exactly what he did.

What led him to leave Ann Arbor for the University of Pittsburgh?

At the time, the University of Pittsburgh wasn't very much of any place. It had a medical school and it had a university, but there were only a couple of people who were full-time faculty at the medical school. The rest were practicing physicians who were teaching on the side. So it did not have anywhere near the reputation that it would later develop. When we came there Jonas found plenty of space at the municipal hospital, but not in prime condition for setting up laboratories. I mean there was a lot of basement space. He really had to start from scratch. He had to do it with a hairpin and Scotch tape.

What was his priority at first?

What he was doing was setting up a laboratory and trying to accumulate staff. The secretary was a young girl, just out of college. When he found she was filing letters under 'L' he started looking for someone else. And that's how he found Lorraine Friedman, who was advertising herself as a Girl Friday, willing to work for an executive. She came to work for him and then together they really set up the lab and began acquiring technical staff to carry out experiments, and eventually built an animal laboratory.

What brought him to polio?

As I recall it, a number of months after he got there, and began setting up the lab, he began talking about the fact that there was going to be a search for identifying the strains of polio virus and that that's what he was going to embark on.

Talk about his novel approach to problems.

It falls into two categories. One is that he was a perfectionist—things had to be done correctly. His approach to problem-solving on the domestic front is well illustrated in a very vivid memory of mine. We lived in Wexford, in the country, when he was doing the typing program. He decided one day to clean the stove. It was a gas stove and we were renting the house. And I'm very tidy, I'm perfectly clean about the front of things, but nothing could interest me less than the back of the stove. Not so Jonas. He took almost the entire day. He pulled it out in the middle of the room, disconnected the gas cord and so forth, and I still recall him cleaning the head of the screws with a toothpick. If it was worth doing, it was worth doing excellently! The other factor was that he had a genius for looking at something and being able to see it in a different relationship than the way it appeared to the rest of the world. It's almost like one of these optical illusions: when you look at it and you see one thing, and then if you look at it long enough the other thing comes out into the foreground. Well, it was a little bit that way with him. It was a combination of an extremely logical mind with these intuitive flashes.

Tell me about his confidence in the possibility of a vaccine.

I think he always had faith in what the outcome would be. Certainly, once the typing program was finished and he embarked on the other, I don't think he ever had any doubt. I think his confidence was supreme. Not in himself, but his confidence in the fact that there had to be an answer to this. And if one approached it in the appropriate way, the answer would reveal itself. As I say that, I can almost hear

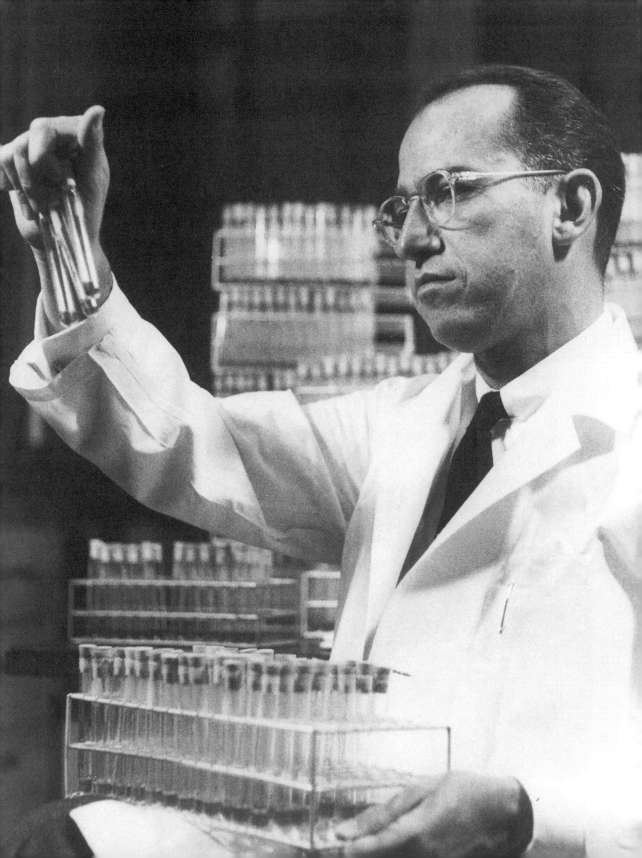

him saying it. That was his style of speaking: 'The answer would reveal itself.' I never doubted him. If he had come home one day after the vaccine, after the field trials and everything, and said, 'I have the cure for cancer,' it would never occur to me to doubt it.

How did he go from the typing program to actually pursuing a prevention of polio?

As Jonas was doing the typing program, his mind must have been leaping ahead to: if this is done, and we type this, then it makes sense that we will be able to do something with this now: 'What approach can we use, having identified these strains of virus, to make this into something that could be eventually useful prophylactically?'

What do you remember about the first vaccine?

When Jonas was first sure about the vaccine he brought it home. He came home, and must have said, 'I've got the vaccine, we're ready.' I remember that the three kids and I were lined up in the kitchen. Now this would be a four-year-old, a seven-year-old, and a ten-year-old lined up and me at the end. I think he gave it to himself first, he gave it to me, and he went down the line and gave it to the kids, and that was all. It was just a piece of what happened during that day. And it really didn't occur to me, never occurred to me, this is a historic moment, or someday will be perceived as an historic moment, not at all. It was just, you know, the guy in the family—my husband, their father—coming home and saying, after all a physician, 'It's time you got a shot,' period. And I had absolutely no doubt that this was an appropriate thing for him to do. It never occurred to me that anything would be wrong, or we could get an effect or something of the sort. It was as to be expected as putting the cat out the door.

Can you tell me his thoughts, anxieties in the first human trials?

I don't recall any ambivalence, because I think Jonas always had his goal in mind. It

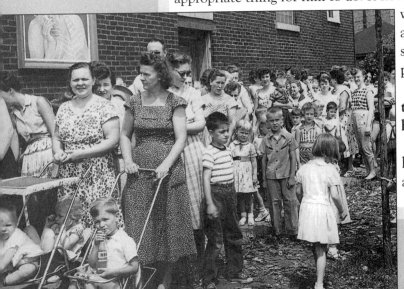

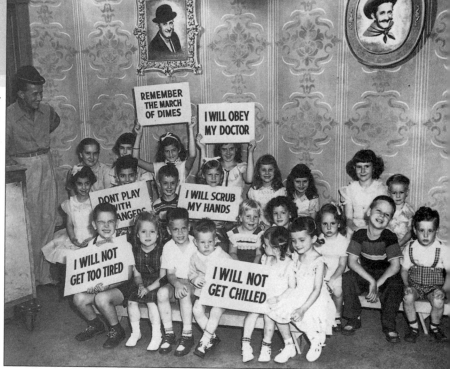

was always framed for him. The perturbations, if there were any, were around the details: 'How many nurses do we need? How many needles do we need? How are we going to line the kids up?' He would have had a say in all of that. That was part of his perfectionism. It all had to be right and he had to know what was going on. So I don't remember any ambivalence on his part about that. When I look back on that I think he should've been very excited. And I think he was excited and stimulated that finally there was going to be a trial in human beings. I'm sure that he did not have any doubts about the fact that it would be okay. With all the confidence and assuredness that Jonas had, it must have caused him some thought, and a small amount of anxiety, at any rate. And after the kids at the Watson Home were inoculated, waiting to see if someone had goofed somewhere, if something was not going to go correctly. Largely because this was a kind of a global anxiety, it wasn't pinpointed on anything specific.

Address his reaction to society's fear and its effect on his research.

I think that the societal fear of polio affected his research, in the sense that that's the motor that was driving him. His determination to do something, to alleviate that fear, the necessity for that fear, the cause of that fear, was always foremost in his mind. There's another factor in there, that is the effect of that societal incubator on the infantile paralysis foundation, on the March of Dimes foundation. That societal pressure generated pressure on the foundation, which

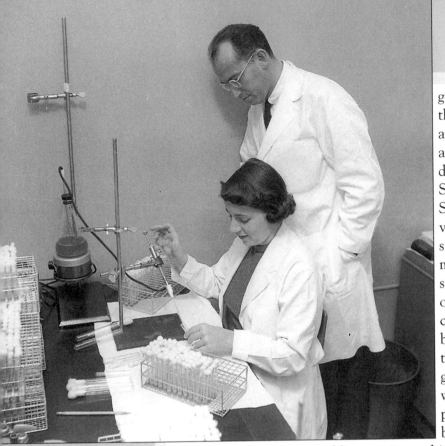

generated pressure on the typing program to be accelerated, and eventually the vaccines to be developed, both the Sabin vaccine and the Salk vaccine. But in my view no external pressure could possibly match the internal pressure under which Jonas operated. He had decided that there ought to be a polio vaccine and that that's what he was going to do. And that was his mission at that point and it was going to be accomplished.

Can you discuss the public reaction to his research?

I remember him going on the radio and speaking about it. I think perhaps he was trying to slow the public down in its expectations. That did not bespeak a lack of confidence on his part at all, but took into account that if the expectation level was rising that high, that it was something that would backfire on the public itself, that they would be disappointed. I'm really not sure that he was thinking about it in personal terms of his reputation. I think he was thinking of it more in terms of it not being a healthy way to deal with this because, as with a disease, if you don't do something to slow it down, it would take over. The expectations would take over and could not possibly be met. Expectations have a way of flying out the window.

What are your memories of Basil O'Connor, then president of the March of Dimes?

Basil O'Connor was an unusual man. He used to speak about the fact that he came from Boston, not from the lace curtain Irish, but from the shanty Irish. He had gone to Dartmouth, and taken his law degree. And he was a very controlling person; very directive is probably better than controlling. And he was extremely determined. He was an intelligent man. He was also a man who very much wanted things to be his way. His influence on Jonas was a very strong one because he was a good politician and he knew there would be plenty of scientific politics. If you think the movie business, or industry, or anything that you could name is a jungle, in terms of people surviving and fighting, academia has it over everything, and research probably more than that. O'Connor knew that and he took that in hand, and he was extremely supportive of Jonas.

On a personal level Jonas was very likely to bow to O'Connor's wishes. Not at all in the scientific realm, but in other areas Jonas was apt to defer to Basil O'Connor's wishes and demands, because in my view O'Connor had an expectation that when he spoke he would be obeyed. He would ask Jonas, for example, to come down to Warm Springs so he could talk with him about important things, but also so that they could play golf, or go to Florida or someplace else. And Jonas would do this, and sometimes it would cut into his lab time, or whatever else he was doing. It was not always appropriate, really. It would've been possible for Jonas to simply say, 'Sorry, Doc, I can't do it.' And O'Connor would have taken that. I know from personal experience with O'Connor that if he asked for something, and the answer was 'no,' and you said 'no,' that was all right with him. He, as many strong people do, respected someone else who would take a stand about something. [But] it was important to Jonas not to have O'Connor's disapproval. So he would defer to him. And O'Connor liked it that way. And it made life simpler.

What was it like being part of one of the great medical discoveries of the twentieth century?

It's very hard to convey to other people, but the kids and I and Jonas lived on a day-by-day basis. One day this happened, one day that happened, then there would be the next day, and the kids would go to school, and then they had a vacation, or whatever might be happening. Now, looking back on it, it sounds ridiculous to say this. Here was

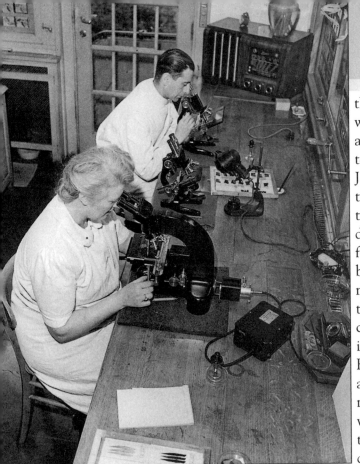

this thing with global potential—which was fulfilled later—and here I am talking about the kids having to go to school. That's the way life was. For Jonas there was obviously a larger picture, which he would come home and talk about, but in a sense it was academic [to me] only because I took it for granted. When the field trials became the next step, that was in the nature of things. It should proceed that way because what was more logical? Here was the vaccine. The experiments had been done at the Watson Home. So I don't think there was an awful lot of discussion about it. My memory of it is of an atmosphere where he would come home and say this and I would say, 'Gee, that's great, dinner's almost ready.' But the 'that's great' was sincere, not dismissive. It would be, 'But of course, one expects this.'

How did Jonas react to the aspersions that were cast on his ideas and work?

Jonas would notice those things of course, and sometimes his feelings must have been hurt by them. But again, because of his internal set, because of his confidence and his knowledge that all the steps he had taken were careful and hedged about with all the appropriate cautions, I don't think that those aspersions touched where he lived as a scientist. They touched where he lived as a human being, because, again, approval was certainly important to him. And the disapproval or the withholding of approval, by fellow scientists was not a happy situation. But I think his inner certainty, that this would be demonstrated, Q.E.D., at a certain point, carried him through that with a degree of, 'if not patience, endurance.'

What are your personal memories of the announcement of the vaccine in Ann Arbor, and its aftermath?

We had no premonition, no idea of what was going to happen—and that includes Jonas—no idea whatsoever. Here we are, a couple of parents taking three kids on their first plane ride. We went there [to] listen to the reports at Rackham Auditorium, and then the next day we would turn around and come back home. We didn't get out of there for five or six days. It was unbelievable when they had to send for Tom Coleman, who was the PR man for the University of Pittsburgh, to come out in a hurry. That the reporters would swarm around and want to talk to us was completely unexpected. And a lot of it was simply about making sure that the kids looked okay, if they were going to be in some sort of photographic thing, that they didn't do anything that was untoward, keeping them entertained. This was hardly a normal vacation for them. As far as the report in Rackham, my memory is that I listened to what Tommy Francis was reporting with one ear, and the other ear and mouth were on quieting Jonathan down, or answering something that Peter was saying, or telling Peter and Darrie to get separate or whatever the thing may be. It's wise to remember that in 1955 society was not the same as it is now in relation to publicity and the media. Not everybody had a television set. There was not the expectation, prior to the event occurring, that everybody would know about it, that everybody would be tracking it, that there would be a barrage of publicity. The people in the media knew that, but the general public did not know that. Therefore there was not the same kind of expectation.

So this burst on the world like a nova. And it burst on us somewhat in the same way because we didn't have any idea that this would cause the kind of repercussions that it did. And as you know, many times it has been said that Jonas became a kind of a folk hero overnight. And there we were, enclosed in Ann Arbor. We just had to take things as they came—interview after interview after interview, and photograph after photograph. And when we got home, it was a little bit different from what it had been when we left. When we got home, the world had changed. And I must say, from our point of view, not for the better. It started with us being met at the airport with a limousine, the first time any of us had ever been in a limousine, and with my asking the chauffeur, please—there was a police escort—to make sure that there were no sirens sounded. And I recall vividly that we lived on a one-way street, and this limousine driver and the police who were on motorcycles were intent on going the shortest way, instead of around the block. So we arrived at the house coming up the street the wrong way, which I recall absolutely horrified me. It was a terrible thing to do. And there was a policeman patrolling up and down the street. I could not understand why. The kids were kind of fascinated by the whole thing. We walked in the house and I remember, the first thing I said was, 'That cop has to leave. What are people going to think?' They'll think the house is about to be bombed. And who's going to bomb the house of somebody that had just found the vaccine that's going to keep their kids from having polio? Why do we need this particular attention? Looking back on it, I think they were probably concerned about the press and so forth, but they were not invasive and did not come into the house.

But things were different. The first thing that happened was that Jonathan, who was age five at the time, walks into the house, and after he puts down his things, goes over to the phone and calls his friend Billy. And both Jonas and I hear him saying, 'Hi Billy, I'm back from my vacation and I'm famous and so is my dad.' We thought, well, that just about says it. [There was] a slew of mail awaiting us. I can recall vividly Jonas and I sitting on the bed opening one letter after another and the letters ranged from: 'This is a wonderful thing, God bless you,' to letters from people who had had polio in the family and who were expressing gratitude for the people who would not get it, to letters from people who themselves had been victims of polio who were writing and so generously saying—I remember how touched we were by the generosity of their saying—'It was too late for me, but it is wonderful that it will be there for other people.' And those letters, every one of those, got answered. Jonas drafted a letter, and it had to be sent to the printers. The mail kept coming for a long, long time. And that was really more gratifying to Jonas and to me than all the celebrity feedback that we had. Not that celebrities weren't sincere, but celebrities have a stake in acknowledging the things that happen. It makes them look good, if I may say that in my usual cynical way. The people you would meet on the street or in the store, in the restaurant, what have you, have no such stake in it. This came from the heart, this came from recognizing Jonas and coming up and being almost wordless sometimes. Or saying to me, 'Aren't you proud of him?' Or occasionally kissing his hand. When, in 1957, we went to the international polio conference in Geneva, we went to a shoemaker who did a double take when he recognized who this was. He just poured out his gratitude. That incident particularly was very meaningful to us. We were

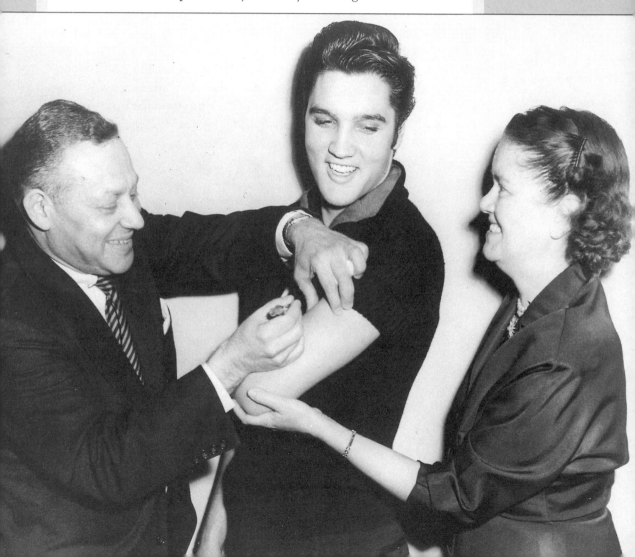

halfway around the world, the language is foreign, and here this man comes up and shares with us what was in his heart. When I was by myself, I would get clerks in department stores who would see my charge card and know my name, saying things to me about it. It still happens.

Can you tell me how the Cutter incident affected Jonas?

That was really a blow. That was a very difficult time for all of us, certainly for Jonas, because everything had gone swimmingly up to this point and I think it was doubly, triply, manifoldly harder for him because he knew from the beginning this should not have happened. This is not the fault of the vaccine or the protocol for manufacturing it. This has to be a glitch somewhere that's a human error. But knowing that could not mitigate the effects of having certain people saying or having the attitude of, 'Well we expected this,' 'We knew from the beginning something would happen.' I'm not talking about the public, I'm talking about some people in the scientific communities. It took some scurrying to do this and some persuading to make sure to track down what had happened, and why it had happened, and how it had happened. Needless to say, it did not happen again, but it took an emotional toll.

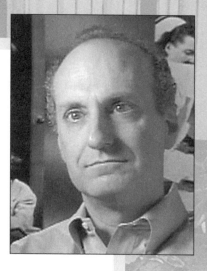

Darrell Salk, M.D.

Darrell Salk is the middle son of Dr. Jonas Salk. He also became a physician and has continued his father's work on the benefits of the killed-virus vaccine.

Could you outline the principles of your father's work?

Prior to the work that Jonas and his colleagues did, it was widely believed that you had to have an actual infection, an active infection, in order to develop immunity against a viral disease. Jonas' work with his colleagues established that a non-infectious vaccine can indeed induce immunity against a viral disease in individuals, and that immunity can be long-lasting. Their work also established that in populations a non-infectious vaccine reduced the amount of virus that's circulating. So that even people who are not vaccinated are protected from being exposed, and therefore don't get the disease. This is called the herd effect. The third important principle that was established by Jonas' work was that the immune system is quite complex and serum antibodies, the chemical that flows around in your blood, is not the only measure of immunity. In the case of polio, something that he referred to as immunologic memory is perhaps a more important measure of the degree of immunity. Previous to this time, people had really been thinking only in terms of measuring antibody levels in the blood. And while that's very important, the immune system is more complex than that. A vaccine that induces immunological memory was a new concept in the use of vaccines.

What is the process of immunization?

There are really three basic ways to become protected against the disease and develop immunity. One of them is to get the disease: in this case the virus gets in, grows, your body recognizes it and it doesn't bother the body again. The other two ways involve purposely giving you something. You can use a virus that is weakened. It will grow in the body, it will expose the body to the virus, but it doesn't cause the disease. The other way is to take the organism, the virus, kill it and administer it. So the body sees it, recognizes it, and develops an immune response. So therefore you become protected against the natural disease, should you become exposed to it.

What are the revolutionary aspects in your father's work?

The approach of the virologists at the time was based on experience with previous vaccines. The successful ones were made with living virus particles. One of the major reasons that had to happen was that in order for the body to recognize and respond, it had to have a big enough dose. The only way to get a big dose was to give you something that would grow in your body because we didn't have technology for growing enough virus outside the body. The conventional wisdom in the 1940s was that the only effective vaccines against virus diseases would be vaccines that were made with living, weakened, but living agents that would grow in the body; that in order to have lifelong durable immunity, there was something special about an active infection. Now, Jonas looked at the fact that there were toxoid vaccines: diphtheria, tetanus, pertussis, that were made with non-infectious agents, and he simply said, 'Well, gee, if it works for that, why doesn't it work for viruses?' And he proceeded to use the technology that allowed growing enough virus outside the body, so that you could administer a large enough dose to have an effective immune response.

What is the science that allowed Jonas to get his solution faster?

There were a number of people who were pursuing the idea of inactivated vaccine, or non-infectious vaccines. My father had worked with some of those people. Tommy Francis was one of the leaders in that. In the case of polio the technology that allowed the principle to be applied was the ability to grow polio virus in bottles, outside of monkeys. Before, when you had to grow it in monkeys and it was the only experimental system you had, it was very expensive, very time-consuming, and very difficult work to do. Once Enders, Weller, and Robbins developed the technology for growing the polio virus in bot-

tles, it was possible to grow large volumes, and then to apply the principle of inactivation, or killing the virus effectively, and then to test it
and see whether that material would work in protecting individuals.
The process for developing an attenuated-virus vaccine basically takes
longer, takes more steps to progressively weaken the virus and test it to
see if it still produces an antibody response and is not dangerously
infectious—it grows, but it doesn't cause disease. It's a longer process.
Once you have killed your agent, a lot of the safety questions and
issues go away. It becomes a much simpler process technologically to
move to creating an immune response. What was crucial in Jonas' perspective, at that time, was to raise the question as to whether it really

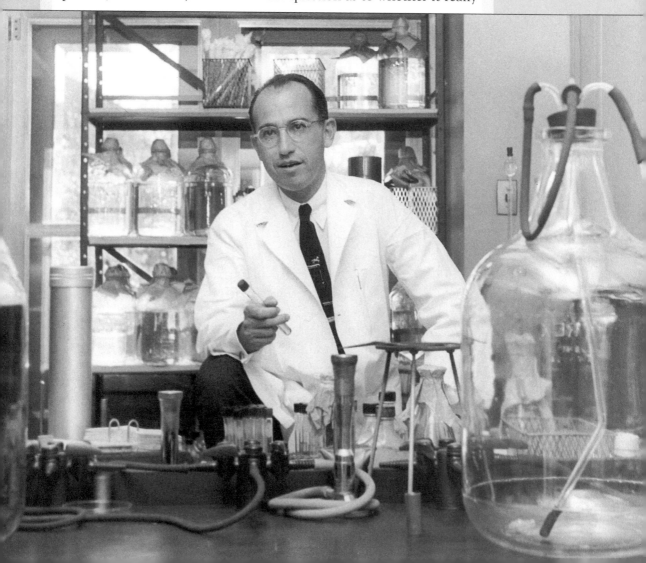

was necessary to have an active infection in order to have an effective immune response. So he and the others working with him could proceed more rapidly toward a vaccine because it was simpler to not have to worry about the safety issues and not have to worry about developing a new type of organism. Instead, you took what you had, you made it safe, and you tested it.

What were the monkey trials all about?

If the only place you can grow the virus is in animals, you have to then take that virus out of the animals and purify it. If you're taking virus from animals' blood, or from animals' nervous systems, there are other materials in it: nervous tissue, body proteins, et cetera. So that what you give as a vaccine has lots of junk in it. Some of the original tests for killed polio virus, vaccine activated vaccines, required growing material in nerve tissue in monkeys, and then purifying that and injecting it into people. As you can imagine when you have a big soup of mashed up brain and you try and clean it and give it to somebody, there's dirt in it, there's lots of other stuff contaminating it. When you have some cells growing in a bottle, and these cells are living in the tissue-culture medium, which you have created and is very pure, all you have to do is take that medium out, filter out the cell material, and you have something that's very pure, and that's what you inject.

Doing research with monkeys is a very complicated business. For instance, you have to have monkeys that are healthy. They have to live in the laboratory for a while to make sure they haven't brought any diseases in. If you're going to grow the polio virus in the monkey unit, you inject it into the monkey. And then you wait and see if the monkey gets sick. This is a process that takes weeks. If you want to compare two viruses, to see if they were similar or not, you'd have to have a monkey that was exposed to one virus, wait for him to get better, give him a big dose from the second virus, and see if he gets sick from that. That tells you whether the two viruses are the same or different. It takes more weeks to do that. And you actually have to use three or four monkeys in a cross experiment.

When Enders, Wellers, and Robbins discovered that you can grow polio virus in the test tubes and bottles in a very clean environment and a very controlled environment, it just changed everything overnight. Jonas sent a technician to learn from Robbins how to do this. She came back and they began to grow the virus in the bottles and in the test tubes. This is really a key change that allowed the development of a non-infectious polio virus vaccine. Because it just speeded up everything almost overnight.

Explain a little bit about the typing experiment.

In trying to understand about the polio disease and to protect against it, one needs to make sure that you're really dealing with all the forms there are. In the 1940s, it was believed that there were three types of polio virus, but it wasn't known if there were more than three or not, or if there were only three. It was important to do typing experiments to establish that type 1, type 2, and type 3 were the only polio viruses out there. If there was a type 4, and if you had a vaccine against the first three types, you'd still get sick with type 4. This was a long slogging that one has to do, testing samples, crossing them to make sure that you've tested everything, and only by doing a large number could you feel confident that there were really only three types. This was the importance of the typing program that was established very early in the 1950s.

There's a reason why your father took on that work with another kind of passion. What was the importance of the typing experiments for him personally?

There was new science in the typing experiments. Jonas actually added some innovations to the use of the monkeys that made the typing experiments more efficient and work better. That is a challenge in and of itself. He had not been work-

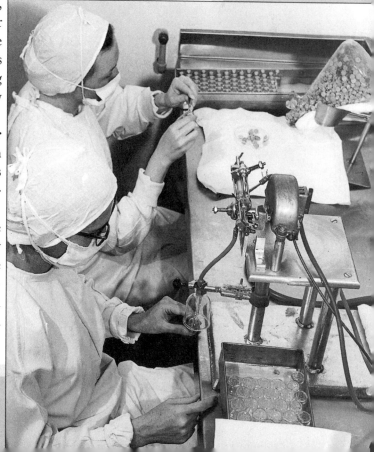

ing with the polio virus before he came to Pittsburgh. And the availability of the typing program and an interest in providing support for that gave him an opportunity to learn something he didn't know about. He'd been working with the influenza virus. For any new researcher, this is a new and exciting challenge. So I think we're looking at a young man who had an opportunity to get involved in a research project, that was something new and exciting and different, i.e., polio viruses particularly, and also be building toward the establishment of a principle that had been in the back of his mind since he was in medical school. And that is, 'Why do you have to have active infection to fool the immune system into developing immunity?'

Describe that scene in your kitchen that day he gave the vaccine to you.

My parents gave the vaccine to the three boys very early. My father didn't know whether it would be effective or not. But he felt that it was safe. He felt that it was something that he wanted to do. For us, it was sort of routine. This was just something that was happening. It was not a mega-event of any kind. Our parents came and said, 'Here, this is something that is going to be good for you' and we were given the vaccine. I think more telling is the fact that the vaccine was used in the laboratory among the workers, because there it was a daily scary thing that they're working with live polio viruses and they have no protection. So the workers, not just Jonas, but all the workers that were there had a vested interest themselves and in the project that they were doing. And once they felt that, as a team, this was safe, and they had an indication in monkeys that it would create an immune response, they protected themselves. They all injected themselves with the vaccine before it was administered to anybody else.

Tell me about the time the announcement was made about the vaccine.

In Ann Arbor there were lots of people around all of a sudden. We had come for what we thought was a vacation. We were going to see where I was born. There were newspaper people around, there were cameras, and from my perspective this was really neat. We ended up getting a police escort on the way home from Ann Arbor and it was a great thrill, very exciting. Better than a roller coaster. Because it was really all part of our lives, basically. Our father was doing research, he had a job and we proceeded. Our life didn't change. People have often asked me, 'What was it like to have a famous father?' Hey—he made me practice the piano when I didn't want to. This was our life.

There have been and certainly continue to be aspersions cast upon your father's work. Talk a little bit about his perception of the naysayers.

What was important to Jonas in the entire process of the development of the polio vaccine, and the many, many years that have gone since then were the basic principles that were involved. He felt strongly that there were important scientific principles to be estab-

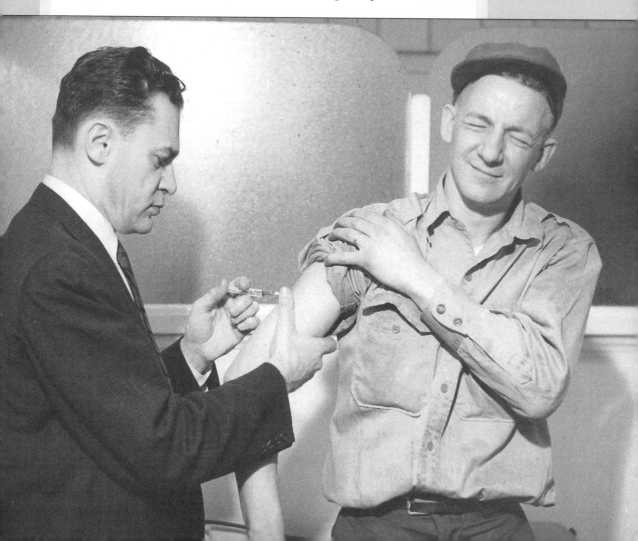

lished, that he and his colleagues had established in their work. It was frustrating to not have those recognized. To not get peer recognition. In a sense, it's not surprising because the kinds of principles they were working on really involved a shift of perspective. And that shift in perspective doesn't happen overnight. The common knowledge at that time among Jonas' peers was that a killed vaccine couldn't possibly work. That belief has continued. There are people that continue to say that today, in spite of the evidence. That can be a very frustrating experience for someone who's trying to get across a principle.

Did he have a response to that? The doubt about his own work?

Jonas received a lot of recognition from the public, which was very gratifying. For whatever reason he did not receive similar kinds of recognition from his peers, which is for anybody a hurtful kind of experience because what drives you is getting recognition that's meaningful to you. As far as our family was concerned, we didn't particularly benefit in a special way from the vaccine. We got no money for it. In a sense we did get a lot of grief from it, because our lives changed. My father, for many years, was unable to pursue the professional and scientific work he wanted to do because of all the brouhaha. So there may very well be a perception among the public that this wonderful thing happened to this family overnight and everything was rosy, meeting the president and all of these wonderful things. It was an ordinary life with these things thrown in on top, which are stressful.

Robert Nix, M.D.

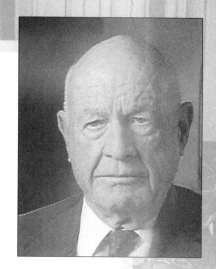

Dr. Robert Nix was the pediatrician for Allegheny County, Pennsylvania in the early 1950s. He was a chief pediatric officer at the D.T. Watson Home where Dr. Jonas Salk first tested the killed-virus vaccine beginning in 1951.

Tell me about your childhood memories of polio.

I grew up in western Pennsylvania. My father was a doctor, a family practitioner. And we lived in a mining town, which was a wonderful experience. We played baseball, we'd swim in the Allegheny River, my younger brother Bill and I. And the dog days in August my mother would say, 'Don't you boys swim in the river, now.' So, we'd play ball, but we'd get so hot, a whole bunch of us would go down to the river, and go skinny-dipping. Come back and play more ball. But that was a real fear in those days. And anytime anybody got sick or had a headache, everybody was really quite frightened. Particularly the mothers. The fathers in the town were miners. Fortunately none of my friends who grew up in the town developed polio. Probabilities are, we maybe had it when we were small, and there was no paralysis.

Tell me about the Watson Home, which became involved with the first human trials of the Salk vaccine.

This home was built by Mr. D.T. Watson, who was a very successful lawyer in Wilson's time, and at one time was ambassador to England. And when he was in England and Switzerland, tuberculosis was the big disease, and he saw these hospitals where they would have children moved out in the sun and be treated. And he decided when he came back that he would build a home and do the same kind of thing that they were doing in Switzerland. He had about three hundred acres up in Wheatsdale, and so he built on that property the D.T. Watson

Home in the late 1920s. It's a brick building, extremely well-built, like a fort. It had lovely rooms and floors and equipment. They had rehab equipment. They had a pool. Back when I got there in 1946, we had about 120 beds, of which eighty or ninety percent were polio. And they had one ward for girls and one ward for boys. And it was as clean as a whistle. Mrs. Lucille Cockler was the superintendent and she was a stickler for cleanliness.

When did you meet Jonas Salk?

I met Dr. Salk first back in 1939 or 1940, when I was a [pediatric] resident in New York and he was at NYU, working with Dr. Francis on the flu vaccine. And he went with Dr. Francis to Michigan and then he came back to Pittsburgh. Well, in 1951 he came down to the Watson Home and asked if he could have the parents give him permission so that he could bleed [take blood from] the children, check them, do the antibodies on them, and try the Salk vaccine on them. As you

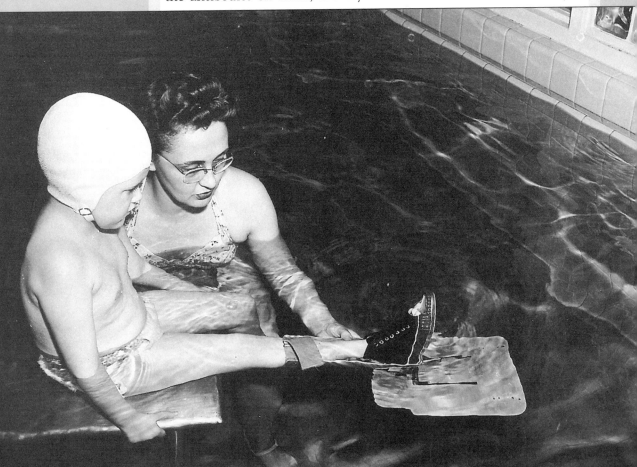

know, polio has three types, and he wanted to determine how much vaccine to give, what vehicle to put it in, whether it be saline, oil, or whatever, and at what intervals the vaccine should be given to give the best antibody response. He came to me and he said, 'Bob can you get me five hundred families? I'd like the children, the parents, the grandparents, and everybody.' I said, 'Sure, I'll get you five hundred.' So I said to Betty Gunnerfinger, who was my nurse, who was my right arm in the office, I said, 'Betty, get ahold of five hundred families,' which she did. The average probably was around six with children and grandparents.

Every Saturday and Sunday, we would stick these people with a needle, take blood, and then give them an injection of the vaccine. He had them come back at two, four, six, and eight weeks. And I would come up every weekend with him. There was lots of action and crying with the small ones. And after he'd done that for two or three months, he came to me again. He said, 'Bob, could you get me five hundred more? I think we could use them.' I called Betty and told her to get five hundred more. And by this time the news was out. People I didn't even know or took care of would call me up and say, 'Dr. Nix, could I get my family included in this study?' Because people were so frightened and concerned about polio, and we had just been through two pretty good epidemics, they would do anything just to get their children in. As a matter of fact, some of the grandparents who had a fair amount of money got their children to come down from New England or wherever they were, to get included in the study. They would bring them back to get their shot and get their blood test done. And there was never a problem, they were so thankful that they were lucky enough to be included in this so-called study. Except some of the children—they were on a schedule to come back to be bled and given an injection in two, four, six, eight weeks—these little rascals would begin to recognize these cards coming in [the mail] and lots of time they'd get the card and hide it because they didn't want the needles.

Let's talk a little bit about Jonas Salk.

Well, Jonas Salk was one of the most unusual men I've ever known. He was a very intelligent man, and he had a lot of empathy. And incidentally, I was good with a needle, but I'll tell you, Jonas Salk was really good with a needle. If he couldn't find a vein, there wasn't a vein around. When he first did his vaccine on the patients in the D. T. Watson Home, he was so concerned, because this was the first time they had done it on many live people. He had done it on some of his staff and his children, I think. But he would go home, and worry, and come back to the home just to check the children and see if everything was all right, that there weren't any reactions. He could have called on the phone and checked, but not Jonas. He had to come back and see it, and do it personally.

He was confident in his vaccine?

Absolutely. It was a killed-virus, so he wasn't concerned so much about that, certainly after the early experience at the Watson Home. I would say around five thousand people were in the study. There were quite a number of people in the medical profession who were not too keen about this set up. [But] Jonas Salk knew the vaccine was good. He knew it was safe. And we who were around realized the same thing, certainly after what he had done with my patients down there. I said, 'Boy, this is the greatest thing since the wheel.' And everybody was just thankful they were able to be in on this.

What was your response on April 12 when they announced the Salk vaccine was 90 percent effective?

Well, when they said that, it was not new. I knew it anyway because we had been doing our study. I knew the vaccine was an extremely good vaccine and a safe vaccine. And quite effective. Frankly, I didn't make too much of it, except that we just talked about it, and said, 'Well, they are finally realizing that the vaccine is really worthwhile.'

Tell me about the followups that were done with the original trial patients.

When the Sabin vaccine was announced and came out in 1963, [Salk] knew it was coming. He wrote to everybody, asking those involved with his original study if they would please hold off 'til he would get a ten-year checkup. He brought a lot of them back in five years and he wanted to have a ten-year followup. And most of the ones that I knew that were on the study didn't take any Sabin vaccine.

Reimert Ravenholt, M.D.

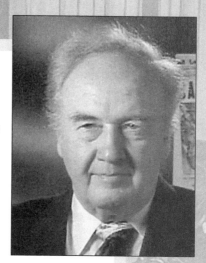

Dr. Reimert Ravenholt was a member of the Epidemic Intelligence Service with the Communicable Disease Unit of the Ohio Department of Health. It was his job to investigate families where multiple members of the family had come down with polio.

What was your first experience working with polio?

I had heard quite a lot about polio, but my first personal, immediate experience with it occurred when I was in my sophomore year at the University of Minnesota Medical School. They had a very large polio epidemic [in the late 1940s]. Three thousand cases or so, and the most severely paralyzed ordinarily ended up at the University of Minnesota Hospital, where they got special care and respirators and so forth. That year the nursing staff got overloaded. They were really stretched, trying to take care of these cases, and they needed to have a little time off at Christmas. I was working my way through so I was happy to have an opportunity filling in, giving nursing care to half a dozen respirator cases, mainly adults. They needed to have the tracheotomy suctioned every half hour, and they needed to be turned every half hour. So it's a very arduous nursing problem. I did that for maybe a week or two during Christmas vacation. It riveted paralytic polio in my consciousness.

When you really got involved with polio was when you joined the Epidemic Intelligence Service. What happened there?

Yes, that was my next major experience, after my internship. In 1953 there was no Salk vaccine available. But everyone was looking for something to protect with and gamma globulin, immune globulin, was

223

traditionally used for a variety of diseases, such as measles and hepatitis. [The question] was whether it would be effective in preventing polio. There was only a limited supply and that year the Center for Disease Control, in conjunction with the state health departments, took control of the immune globulin supply in the country. And the Epidemic Intelligence Service was given the task of developing what was called the National Program for the Evaluation of Immune Globulin for the Prevention of Poliomyelitis. They were giving it, hoping it would prevent polio, but there was no solid evidence for that yet. So it was put under test, with followup. It consisted of studying what happened in multiple-case households. When one case of polio occurred in the household, the person contacted would often receive immune globulin. And if it were effective it would prevent or intensely modify the subsequent cases in the household. The program consisted of evaluation: What happened when household contact cases were given the globulin? I was assigned to Ohio. I would have to get initial epidemiological data and then do very thorough testing of each of the muscle groups to see how much weakness there was, if any. We had had special training in the spring of 1953 in muscle testing, up at Pittsburgh, close to Jonas Salk's operation there. This kept me busy up through the summer of 1953, traveling throughout Ohio, not only to homes but also to the main hospital centers. But the bottom line was that 'passive immunization' was never proven to be useful for that purpose. The difficulties of administering it at the right time to the right person were insurmountable.

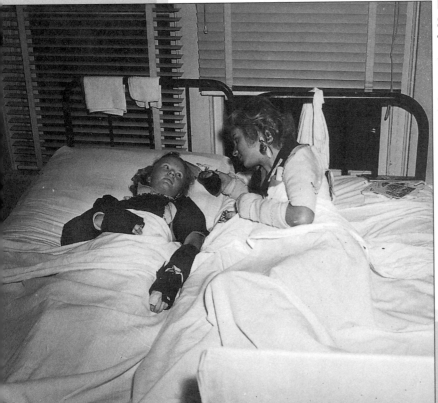

What were your impressions of the public response to polio?

The fear and the interest of the public in immunization prevention was so intense. We don't really see anything that intense anymore. I mean, we have many serious disease problems now. AIDS is a great problem, but it happens to only certain populations, so that the general public is not fearful of AIDS. But at that time in the 1950s polio occurred unexpectedly, hitting adults as well as children out of the blue. And the people were just desperate to get an effective prevention.

Tell me what happened in 1955.

In the late fall of 1953, I transferred from Ohio and was assigned to the Seattle County Health Department and soon became the director of epidemiology and disease control there. 1954 was the summer that the Salk vaccine was tested in quite a few key areas in the United States. We did not participate in the field trial that summer. Then what happened was that the analysis from the collected data from that field trial was done by Dr. Tommy Francis at the University of Michigan on April 12, 1955. And it was transmitted on television and to movie theaters. And indeed here in Seattle myself and many physicians went to one of the theaters to see on the screen the Francis report and the commentary upon it. The report was that the vaccine had proven to be both safe and effective through the field trials of 1954. That indicated that we could indeed go ahead. And we had already planned and arranged to immunize. I had recruited 160 voluntary private physicians to administer these injections, so as soon as we got the word that the vaccine was both safe and effective I went back to my office and telegrammed the National Foundation in New York to ask them, 'When do we get our vaccine?' And they said well, they didn't know exactly but we would be getting our vaccine for Seattle County from Cutter Laboratory in Berkeley, California. Well, I knew something of Cutter because we had purchased the smallpox vaccine, DPT, for the school program here for a number of years. So I telephoned Bill O'Neil [at Cutter], whom I knew, and asked when we would get our vaccine. And he said quite casually over the phone that he'd get it to us as soon as possible, but they had trouble with one lot that they had to throw away. It was several days later that I got a telegram from Cutter that the vaccine supply would be on Western Airlines the next day.

The following day when I got to the office I had another telegram saying that because there was not enough to supply the entire state of Washington, they were diverting the entire supply for Seattle County to Idaho, with its smaller population. About that time a couple of the Cutter detail men took the director of maternal child health, Dr. Wilke, and myself to lunch to discuss vaccine supplies. And in the course of that, one of the Cutter men said, 'Sorry that the vaccine supplies were so tight.' They could not be available to us for personal use. To which I nonchalantly replied, 'The Parke Davis man said he'd give me some vaccine.' I went back to my office and a couple of minutes later a breathless messenger arrived with a dozen vials of Cutter vaccine for Dr. Wilke and myself and other health department personnel. I had an immunization clinic right next to my office there. So I put the vaccine in the refrigerator and at the end of the afternoon, Dr. Wilke came by to get vials of vaccine to immunize his children. And I laughingly told him, 'You go ahead. I'll wait a few weeks. Then I'll immunize my own two children.' But then upon reflection, if I didn't have enough confidence in the vaccine to immunize my own two children, I shouldn't be directing a program that would immunize everybody else's children. And I took one of the vials home with me and I immunized my two children, Janna and Marc, ages four and two, that night. Well it was just three days later that the news came over the wire: Cutter vaccine causing paralytic polio in California and Idaho. I immediately contacted the California health offices and very specifically asked what the lot number was of the offending vaccine. I immediately checked the lot that I had and sure enough it was the bad lot. And indeed my two children that night and for several days were running fevers. But fortunately they had an aborted infection that did not develop paralysis. But that, of course, was somewhat traumatic.

Joseph Melnick, M.D.

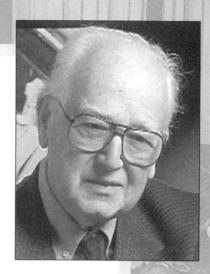

Dr. Joseph Melnick was a scientist at Yale University and was central to the development and testing of the oral polio vaccine. He, and others, worked with Albert Sabin in developing a live, attenuated virus now used in most parts of the world.

How did the public's fear motivate the search for the vaccine?

The polio epidemics in the 1950s were like the AIDS epidemics today. And the reporters picked this up and put this in the papers and people got hysterical about it. Very often when I went to epidemic areas, the first thing that we would do when we'd come to a new city was to meet the reporters. And we'd get off the plane and when all the reporters were down they'd say, 'What are you gonna do?' And we said 'Well, we'd like to go swimming.' And we went swimming in Los Angeles, and the reporters sort of flowed right along. And the community relaxed. Because if the experts went swimming instead of doing whatever they were going to do, the community thought there wasn't much seriousness to what the reporters were writing about.

What happened in the ten years between the Salk and Sabin vaccines?

When the results of the Salk field trials were announced, there was a gap. Some 40 percent of people were not protected with the vaccine. It was 60 percent for type 1, and something like 80 percent for type 2, and the country was relieved. The vaccine protected, but the fact that it wasn't 100 percent didn't make much difference. The fact that it protected was important. But there were a few laboratories that still felt that they'd like to have a vaccine that was 100 percent. Sabin was one of them, our laboratory at Yale was another. We continued to work in developing a live-virus vaccine.

Can you describe your research into the live-virus vaccine?

When I first started to work at Yale on this problem, I was concerned about where the virus existed in nature. And one of the things that was happening was that we were learning that patients had the virus in their gut. And if it appeared in the gut, it would appear in the stools and would be washed away in the sewer system. Now we knew there were more people with the virus in their gut than appeared in the hospitals. So we decided to carry out a study in New York City during periods when there was virus and when there was no virus. And we found that when there was little virus in the community, we could detect virus in the sewage. The virus in the sewage must be coming from the virus that the people were excreting, even though they were not ill. We could determine the number of people that were infected in New York City, and it turned out that there were one hundred people infected for every one that was in the hospital. That immediately told us that the virus belonged to a group of viruses that lived in the alimentary tract of people.

What did that mean to vaccine research?

Well, it tells us that we have to work with the virus so that it can still inhabit the gut, but not the nervous system, which is the target organ for the virus once it gets into the body. The

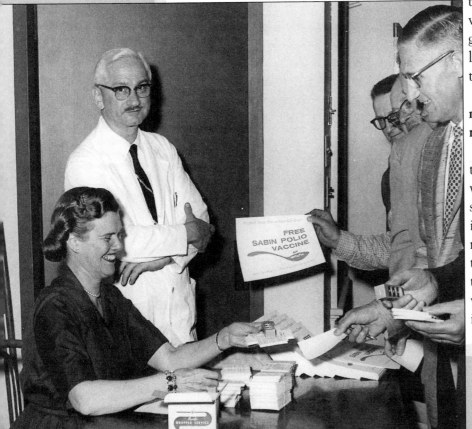

virus doesn't do anything in the gut except to multiply. If we can keep it multiplying, and not producing disease, we have a vaccine because the multiplication of the virus in the gut is enough to prevent the target organ from being infected. In other words, we needed a mutant virus. We knew that they existed in nature. We continued looking for a duplication of what nature did, a virus that would still replicate in the gut and would not allow the target organ, the central nervous system, the brain, the spinal cord, to be infected. And the National Foundation, in order to keep people like Albert Sabin quiet, gave him a substantial amount of money.

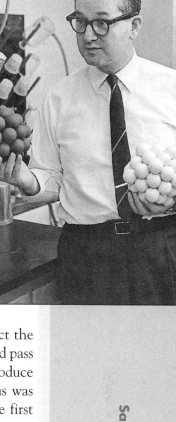

Why couldn't you achieve the live-virus vaccine before Salk's?

Well, it's very hard to do the first experiment on people. You don't want to subject a person to a virus that may infect the target organ. What we were doing was to take a virulent virus, and pass that in animals, and show that it maintained its ability to produce infection in the gut and not the nervous system. But that virus was tested in monkeys, chimpanzees, but not in people. So that the first people who received it were guinea pigs.

Tell me about the field trials in the Soviet Union.

The Soviet Union is a large country, like ours, and was having polio epidemics in the 1950s. And like our country, they had produced the Salk vaccine. But they had difficulty immunizing. I remember that some Russian scientist told me they didn't have enough syringes to distribute the vaccine. So when Albert Sabin came around, and this was a virus that could be given by mouth and not by syringe, the Soviet Union latched onto it and gave it to a large number of people. And the results that were made available to the committee, that I served on at NIH, demonstrated that the Sabin vaccine was one that could be given safely and protected a large number of people.

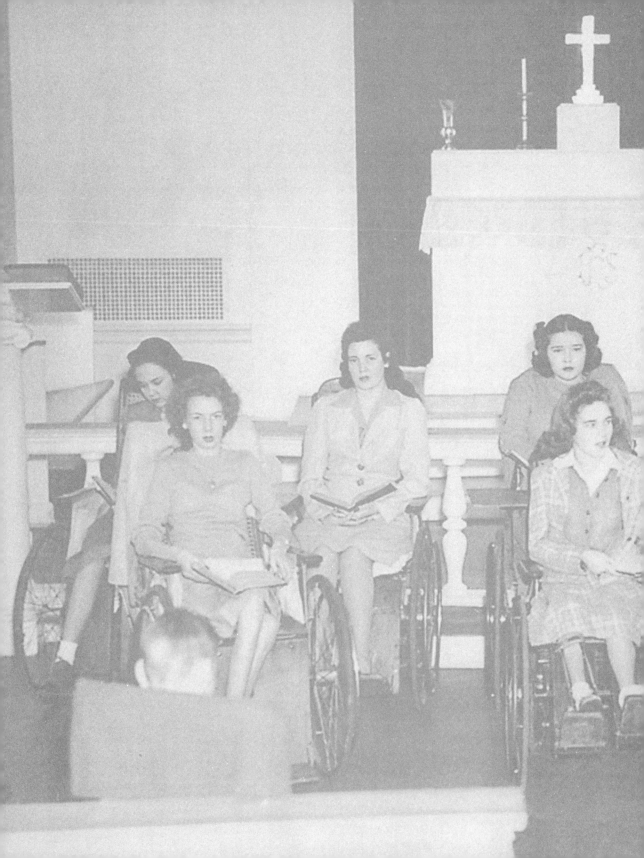

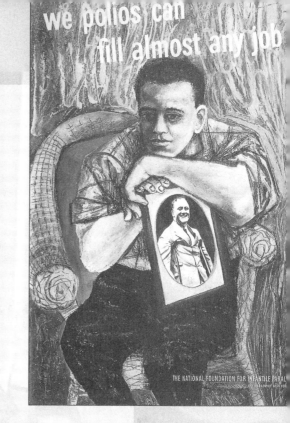

we polios can fill almost any job

THE NATIONAL FOUNDATION FOR INFANTILE PARAL...

Chapter 6

Polio Survivors and Post-Polio Syndrome

Sure, I'd like to walk. You know I never carried my bride across the threshold and I was too big for her to carry me, so that didn't happen. I never carried my child. I never carried a bag of groceries in my life. But I've had a lot of other experiences that other folks haven't had, and so I don't fret about not being able to walk, or not being able to ride a bike, even though that may be kind of interesting again. I have two philosophies that I kind of use: one of them is that life is a deck of cards. You either play them or you throw them in. I think that playing them is better than throwing them in. And the second one is you waste a lot of valuable time sitting around trying to figure out what might have been. You take what you have, and you go with it. And that's what I've done all my life.

—Arvid Schwartz,
polio survivor

231

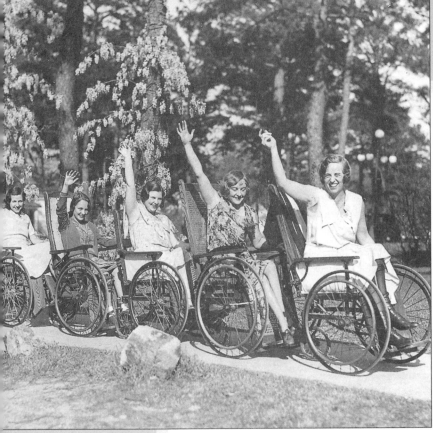

As many as twenty million polio survivors around the world still struggle with the after-effects of polio. For these people, and for all the families of those who suffered or died in the past, the epidemic era never ended.

In the United States alone, there are now approximately 600,000 known polio survivors. Some have lived for decades with varying degrees of disability. Many more thought they had escaped with minimal injury from their bout with polio almost half a century ago, only to discover a new constellation of problems that may be traced back to their initial infection. Over half of the known survivors of the polio epidemics before 1960—several hundred thousand people in the United States—are now experiencing physical difficulties that are related to their original case of poliomyelitis.

The emergence of the late effects of polio was as unexpected as the first epidemics. In the early 1970s, men and women, who thought they had put their polio years behind them twenty or thirty years before, began to report mysterious symptoms that might possibly be related to their earlier disease. Joint and muscle weakness, general fatigue, pain, sleeping problems, increased sensitivity to cold, and difficulty in swallowing and breathing were all reported. What no one knew was whether these were normal signs of aging, a recurrence of the virus, symptoms of some new condition, or a sign of psychological difficulties. Patients were scattered and we had no way of comparing their experiences. Doctors rarely saw enough cases to recognize a trend.

Like polio itself, the various symptoms that have come to be known as "post-polio syndrome" or "late effects of polio" must have existed for decades or even centuries before they were recognized. Once again, it was the mounting number of cases that made the mysterious new condition impossible to ignore. And, once again, the sufferers were forced to confront medical ignorance, social indifference, and the groping mistakes of early therapies that did little to help the problem they hoped to solve.

In 1981, the first grass-roots conference on post-polio syndrome was organized by the Gazette International Networking Institute (GINI). In 1984, the Post-Polio League for Information and Outreach was established. Now known as the Polio Society, with headquarters in Washington, D.C., it serves as an information clearing-house on medical and other health-related issues to both polio survivors and health care professionals. Rehabilitation centers have begun to offer specific treatment for post-polio patients, and doctors have grown more aware of the syndrome and better able to distinguish its symptoms from other medical conditions.

Recognizing the symptoms of post-polio syndrome has been easier than understanding its causes. Although many theories have been offered, from premature aging to psychological difficulty to a recurred virulence of a latent virus, the current consensus of medical opinion is that the many forms of post-polio syndrome all relate to the loss of nerve and muscle function during the original infection. When some motor neurons were destroyed, others developed new terminal axon sprouts to innervate orphaned muscle cells, sometimes growing to a giant motor unit that might innervate as many as ten times its original number of muscle cells. Over time, however, the neuron may not be able to generate new cells fast enough to keep up with the death of older cells, causing a progressive lesion. Alternately, what is know as a fluctuating lesion may occur, caused by a failure in the synthesis or release of the neurotransmitter acetylcholine. In either case, the result is new muscle weakness.

For those who underwent aggressive rehabilitation in the 1940s and 1950s, there is an irony in their new weakness, for it contradicts everything they were taught about the philosophy of recovery. Children who were encouraged to exert themselves beyond the limits of the comfortable or, it seemed at times, the possible, are now discovering that the regained mobility of their youth has led to severe limitations in late-middle age. People who fought to learn to walk and were proud of their strength and mobility now face the bitter possibility that the very efforts that restored their vigor overtaxed their damaged nerves. They are worn out before their time.

One more time, it seems, polio survivors will have to create a new model for disability. The ideal now is not the active overachiever who insists on the value of the struggle and the necessity of independence, but the realist who balances ability and disability, conserving energy for the most precious and necessary activities. The hardest adjustment for those struck by the late effects of polio may lie in learning to accept their limits.

We live in a very different world from the one that greeted the survivors of the 1916 epidemic. New mechanics make possible wheelchairs, scooters, and stair glides powered by computers, by engines, or by very smallest puffs of breath. The iron lung has shrunk to the portable respirator, and orthopedic braces are lighter and more comfortable. Generations of activism for minority rights have laid the groundwork for battles that might otherwise be too difficult for people of diminished strength. The home and workplace can be modified to permit continued activity within the range of personal function. We know a great deal more about how to manage pain, both through medication and psychological support, and through evolving techniques of physical therapy and exercise.

New societal understanding of the vast capacities of those with physical limitations, backed up by new laws that demand access for the disabled, mean that those suffering from the late effects of polio will not be relegated to the proverbial back rooms of an earlier age. Still, it is hard to wake in the morning and realize that the nightmare monster of polio has come back to stalk us once again.

Voices
Richard Owen, M.D.

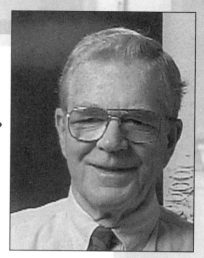

Richard Owen was twelve years old when he contracted a bout of polio that left him without the use of his legs. Since, he has become a physician specializing in the treatment of individuals with the current-day effects of polio known as Post-Polio Syndrome.

Think about the first moment in your life when you realized something was wrong.

It was the morning of October 3, 1940. I was twelve years old. I had gone back to bed with what I thought was a cold with a fever, and I was happy because I was getting out of school. I fell asleep and an hour later I woke up. I was getting out of bed and fell to the floor, and I couldn't get up. I thought something was awfully wrong, but I had no idea what it was. It was just a mysterious experience to me. I had never known people before who were paralyzed or weakened, so I didn't understand that. And also I was raised in a medical family, so I had the feeling it was something fixable because everything else had been fixable. I remember my mother coming up and helping me back into bed, and then she called my father, and then the next thing I knew an ambulance was there. And they took me to the Indiana University Hospital, and put me in isolation.

What did you know about polio at the time?

Franklin Roosevelt was President since 1932 and he had been sort of the focal point for the March of Dimes. I had seen him in 1936, when he visited Indiana University Medical Center. He drove up for the therapeutic pool, which was interesting because later I was in that pool. Roosevelt was in an open car and they had built a ramp for his car to come up. I knew he needed this ramp to get up and he didn't get out of his car. So I had that vision of a person with polio. Unfortunately, or perhaps fortunately, my mind really didn't connect the thing that I had with him, because he had 'infantile paralysis,' and I had a disease with a long name that I didn't quite catch when they put me in the hospital.

Did you have any fear of polio?

No. Mostly the children who had polio were put off in crippled children's schools. So there was nobody with a visible physical handicap in any school I had ever attended.

What were your thoughts when you went to the hospital?

Initially I was rather dazzled by the attention because, being a teaching hospital, there were the physicians and residents and interns and medical students, and the room was packed with people, or at least it seemed to me. I was lying out flat, and there was mumbling and a use of words I didn't understand, but I was sort of swept along by attention. So I wasn't particularly experiencing fear, except when they started to examine my legs and found that I had no movement. My legs were very tight and painful, so I had an additional fear that maybe they were going to take it beyond the point of pain that I couldn't tolerate well.

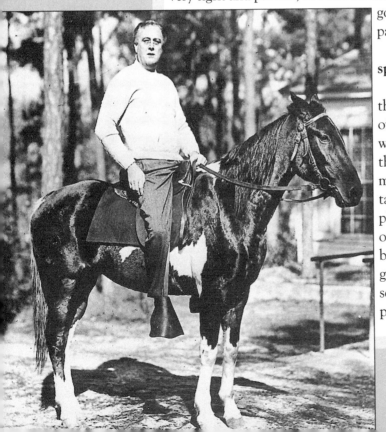

What about when they did a spinal tap?

I became quite nervous about the event. Up until that time I sort of had some sense that something would be done, and I'd be out of there. In fact I remember asking my mom if I would not have to take dancing lessons, and if I could play football when I got out. And of course, not realizing that probably was a painful question to her, I got permission to skip dancing lessons and piano lessons and I could play football.

What was going on with your parents during this time?

I saw my father daily because he was a physician at Indiana University, so he would come in. I had no idea how he was feeling, I really didn't. His bedside manner was so smooth that he'd look at my chart and see what my fever was doing. He'd squeeze my toe and say, 'Can you feel that?' But I'd seen him do those things with other people when he was in a physician-patient relationship. That was just part of his style. So I felt no particular fear on his part. My mother was very supportive and came to the hospital almost every day, brought some of my favorite things along, brought a teddy bear that I had, and a football. So I slept with these two familiar things. And also it was the time of Wendell Willkie's campaign, and she brought me a picture of him so I started collecting Willkie buttons. And that sort of was a distraction for me. [She] brought me Coca-Cola, which was probably a mistake because it added to my increase in weight over a period of nine months in which I was down flat. I had an older brother and older sister who were kept at home in quarantine. And that was her additional responsibility.

What was the community's response to the fact that you had polio?

Well, it was kind of disquieting because my mother got a number of calls from people that questioned whether there was one awful sin besides original that happened, that caused this bullet out of the blue to strike my family. That bothered her a great deal and yet she was a strong person and was able to fight back quite well.

While you were in isolation in the hospital, what were the attitudes of the doctors and nurses toward you?

For some odd reason I looked upon the whole interaction as sort of a social thing. It was a pleasant group of people that would come in to see me. All very supportive and smiling and talking about how Indiana University did in football, and how the Indianapolis Indians, the baseball team, was playing at the time. Here again, I wasn't overburdened with fear for some strange reason. During the early part, I think, I had episodes of being so sleepy during the day and so wide awake during the night. I might have been groggy enough during the day that some of the things that should've bothered me didn't.

What kind of treatment did you get?

The treatment at that time was immobilization. So I was given a pair of things called Toronto's splints, which were leather-covered gadgets with padding. And those were used to keep my legs in what was called the neutral position. That was the main thing, inactivation, which was probably the weirdest experience of all because I'd never been inactive before.

Can you talk about the day you were told you could get out of the hospital?

I was very delighted and I hadn't considered up to that time anything, but that I would be back to normal the moment I got out of the hospital. At that time you always thought that hospitals were places you stayed in until you got well. And that was my vision, that I would get out and suddenly, miraculously return to normal. Now that sounds bizarre to me, that I should have had that feeling. But that was my thought, that I would go home and get on my bike.

What actually happened?

I went home with a frame with canvas on it and with these leather splints that was put up on blocks in my bedroom, and that's where I lay for the next eight months. The therapist came out from Indiana University Medical Center and would carry out what was called 'range of motion,' which was just a gentle sort of stretching of tight muscles. But there was no particular emphasis on trying to re-educate the muscles to work. And it was a very passive experience. I just was a passive receiver of exercise, nothing was demanded of me.

At home, what was your relationship with your friends?

Initially my friends came often, and then they stopped coming so frequently. I think it was partly that they ran out of things to talk to me about. I joined Boy Scouts just before I got polio. And the scout master and the scout troop came, and they gave me an honorary first-class badge. And they all sent me notes and then didn't come anymore.

Can you tell me about those months that you laid in bed?

Three hours a week I had tutoring. To get through part of the seventh and part of the eighth grade with only three hours of schooling suggests that maybe there's extra time in school that is unnecessary. During the mid part of the day, when my brother and sister were away, I would listen to soap operas. I listened to all of these things. I can remember Ma Perkins and My Gal Sunday. I would have the therapy three days a week. A visiting nurse would come one day a week and that was about it. I think our minister would come, and periodically some other friends of my parents.

Can you tell me about the image of yourself lying in bed?

It was a bizarre image. The frame was made so that my bottom hung out. That was to take a bed pan. I used a bed pan and urinal at that time and had bed baths, which were brought to me as a basin of warm water with soap. I had a routine wash down, which was an interesting anatomical exercise because I'd wash my face first, and then wash all the parts of my body I could reach, and then usually my mother, or the nurse, would come wash my legs. My head was propped up enough so I could eat regularly, and eat excessively for someone not exercising.

Can you tell me about the day you got up?

I was readmitted to Indiana University Hospital and started with braces on both legs. And I was brought up to parallel bars, and brought to a stand by three people getting me off the frame and up. So that was

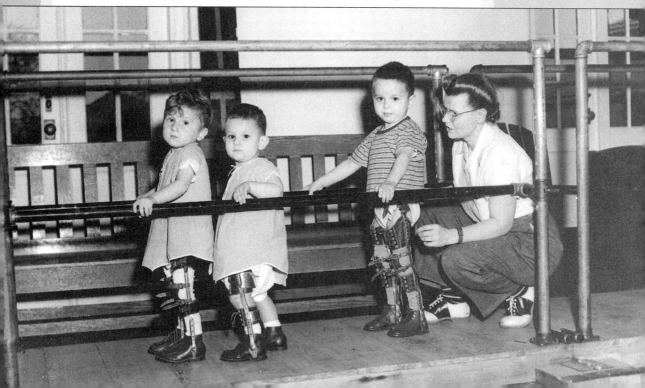

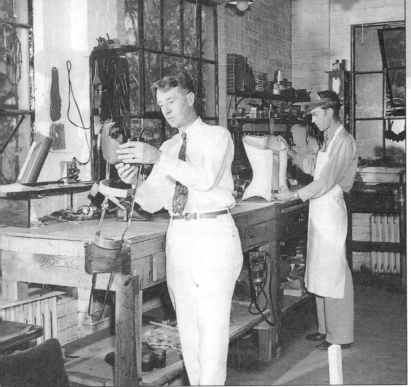

my first experience. I'd grown eight inches and fifty pounds while I was lying down. All of a sudden my center of gravity was far above where it had been before. The ground looked so far away and my legs were so unbendable. It was a very frightening thing. It was almost as if I didn't want to do it because of the increase in height. Then, after they started me on that, they built me long leg braces with a pelvic band to hold my trunk upright, and I got a brace for my right leg as well, so that the total weight was fifteen pounds of bracing. I hadn't used the muscles that were supposed to move that equipment in so long that it was very difficult to get an idea of how I was going to move along. I was given two crutches and learned what was called gait training, which was mainly learning how to swing all that apparatus through on crutches.

Tell me why you laid there for nine months.

They told me that the virus would remain active for about nine months and could make me more paralyzed than I was. That was hard for me to understand because I couldn't imagine being more paralyzed than not being able to move my legs or my abdominal muscles, so that didn't make an awful lot of sense to me. But it was apparently some concept of viral activity that wasn't clear to them, and wasn't clear to me, and I couldn't understand why I was gotten up at nine months while maybe some others earlier and some later.

Two years after you first contracted polio, you had treatments. Tell about that.

The staff at Indiana University had trained with Sister Kenny up in Indianapolis. They became very excited about the concept of Sister

Kenny, who at that time had emphasized flexibility and motor control rather than bracing and strengthening. So the staff at Indiana University was rather excited to find some pleasant compliant person to start that on, and they chose me. It forced me out of school for a semester and during that time I was taken to the University Hospital. And I would have hot packs put on for about thirty minutes at a time, and then removed, and then put back on, and removed, and then stretching exercises two or three times a day.

Tell me what it was like to go back to school.

I had returned to school after my gait training. It was a most bizarre experience because I had grown a lot and I hadn't seen the majority of my classmates. My best friend was a year older than I, so I hadn't noticed the gradual changes in him. To lie down at age twelve and come back at age thirteen was an astounding time period because the girls had changed so much and so unexpectedly for me. No one had introduced me to the fact that they might have changed. And all of the boys were bigger, and they all had deeper voices, and I was getting one too.

How did they accept you on those braces and crutches?

I'm not really sure. I think it was such a strange event for them because it was unusual for a child, with a physical disability as severe as mine, to be integrated in a regular classroom. I came back to a group of people who had known me, and here I was on two crutches and lugging a fifteen-pound brace with me. The teachers were extraordinarily marvelous to me, which was a disadvantage for me then, and in high school, because I was looked upon as something special. And I'm sure that I was given grades that I oftentimes didn't work for, didn't deserve.

How did you handle the physical challenges when you got to college?

The campus at Indiana University is very hilly. It was part of my desire to be entirely normal. I was on crutches part of the time because I had one of my ankles fused during that time. Using crutches, I was able to zip around a little faster. At that time they had no idea about wheelchairs and most wheelchairs were not easy to move about any place anyway. I found that there were many stairs, no elevators. And the lack of a sense of need to accommodate people with disabilities was so great that after two years I decided that I better not continue there.

How did you get into medical school?

I decided rather early that I wanted to go to medical school primarily because of my experiences as a patient. My dad was a doctor, his father was a doctor, and *his* father was a doctor. So we went back a long time in history as physicians. There was something about the applicability of the knowledge of biology to problem-solving that made it exciting to me. I loved nature and I loved zoology and it seemed like this would be one place where I could do all of those exciting things, plus make a living. When I applied to medical school, I found that many schools felt that they couldn't accommodate a person with a physical disability. In fact, at the medical school that I [eventually] made it into, the admissions director felt that it would be impossible for me to make it through medical school. That was one reason why I was all the more determined to make it in. I went to him and I told him that I'd already hiked mountains in Canada, and I swam regularly. I felt that I was in good enough physical condition to do this. And he said, 'Well, how about stairs?' So for the first two years of medical school I climbed up and down the stairs to prove that I could do that too. But it was difficult because there was no sense of architectural accommodations for disabled people.

Tell me about when the vaccine came out.

I was at Warm Springs, Georgia, for a course in rehabilitation of people with polio. And it was on April 12, the anniversary of Roosevelt's death, when the information was released. It had been kept a secret primarily I think for publicity purposes. The information had largely been gathered as to the effectiveness of the Salk vaccine. But the release of the information was on April 12, and we, by chance, were in Warm Springs for this review conference. The excitement of the place was just immense and the media people were all down interviewing patients and finding out how thrilled everyone was. And, as you can imagine, to a person who had polio

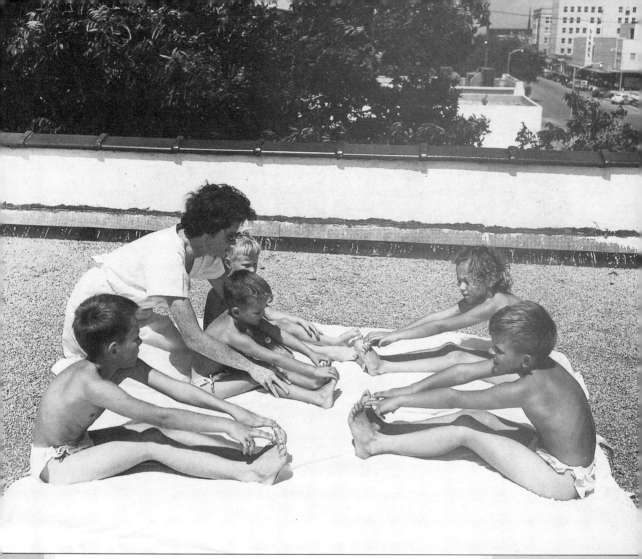

and who was in that setting, there must've been a feeling of the
thrill for the fact that this disease wouldn't happen ever again. That
was what it seemed the message was.

But how did you feel as a person who had polio?

I was thrilled too. The fact that I had polio in a strange way never
has bothered me long-term. I think it's been one of the things that has
shaped my life and career, and that if I wouldn't have [had it] I don't
know what would have been my life activity or interest. The fact that
polio's largely preventable, and that there's been no cases in the Western hemisphere since 1991, is really very thrilling.

Can you tell me about the last epidemic? Now you were seeing it, not as a patient but as a professional.

In 1959, in Minnesota, we had an epidemic in which we had one hundred patients that had acute paralytic polio. We had that over a two- to three-month period of time. And it was very difficult to bring the organization back to the level for the necessary management of an acute infectious disease. After actually changing into a rehabilitation hospital, we were treating people primarily with spinal cord injury, stroke, and head injury, with only a few people left from the polio years who were still hospitalized. So all of a sudden we were taking care of people who were acutely ill with fever, with headache, with tight, sore muscles, with paralysis; and needing tight spinal taps, needing isolation, and needing the rehabilitation techniques that Sister Kenny originally introduced in 1940 to the United States. This was a very difficult re-adjustment for our staff. For instance, it had been a long time since I had taken care of acutely ill patients, and suddenly I was one of the two full-time medical staff at Sister Kenny.

Did these patients bring back things from when you were a patient?

It should have, but it didn't, and I think it's partly that this was a period in which I was working with a cloak of denial that protected me from thinking about these things. I realized that I had a bond or some sense of relationship to the people. And the patients, and the parents had some feeling that perhaps I would understand what they were going through. In many ways I had some sense of remoteness from that. That sounds kind of strange, but I think that was my way of getting on through and doing the job.

Mark Sauer

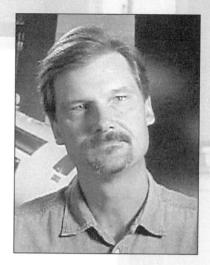

Mark Sauer contracted polio when he was six years old in 1958 during the last major epidemic in Detroit. He was left unimpaired by his bout with polio. He has become a journalist in San Diego.

Can you describe the moment when you realized something was wrong with you?

I was six years old. We had spent weekends that summer going out to a local park called Kensington. My sisters and I and my folks went every Saturday. We would play in the water and picnic. It was just a ritual that whole summer. Toward the end of the summer, it may have been Labor Day weekend, we were out at Kensington and as we got up to leave that day, I got very dizzy and disoriented. I actually bumped right into a parking sign and my parents obviously noticed that something was wrong. I got in the car and I was quiet, sleepy, not feeling at all well. I got home and my folks didn't think anything of it. Kids, they get sick and snap out of it an hour later. So we decided to go to the drive-in movies that night, which is another thing we did quite often in those days. We loaded up the bottles of soda pop and got blankets in the back seat. And in the back seat I got violently ill and began vomiting and had sweats and a fever, and my sister also was vomiting. The folks took us home and they were quite concerned. They watched me all night long, and that night I was quite ill. The next morning they took me to the emergency room at Ford Hospital in Detroit. They thought I had the flu or a bug or something going around that particular week and were concerned with the start of school. They really were caught off guard when the physician on hand said that it was probably polio, given the symptoms and the fact that there were an enormous number of cases that summer. I learned in later years that

that was the last big epidemic in Detroit. And of course the vaccines had already been introduced and had started to take hold. In fact, I had gotten a vaccine with my sisters early that summer.

When the physician used the word polio, my mother looked over to my father and I immediately saw tears welling in his eyes. It hadn't occurred to them at that point that this was anything other than a typical childhood illness, maybe a stomach bug. They simply were overcome because polio was such a horrible dread to any parent at that time. It's almost a physical reaction, when you heard that word at that time. It's a simple word, but it carries such connotations for a parent in the 1950s.

What happened at the hospital?

My sister was diagnosed with a much milder case and sent home. I was admitted. The hospital at that time was dealing with an epidemic. There were kids on gurneys in the halls, there were kids in every spare space they had, all polio victims. I had an isolation room because my case was considered to be quite contagious and advanced. Being six years old, I was old enough to remember and start forming some lasting memories. I was past that childhood amnesia age, three, four, or five years old. Some of the earliest memories I have had to do with that stay in the hospital, that bout with polio. I remember right at the time of being admitted that my parents were in the room. They immediately decided to give me a spinal tap and the nurse was preparing me for it, and she gave me her four fingers and had me clutch them in my fist. I wrapped my little fist around her four fingers and kind of stared at her fingertips as they had me on my belly and were inserting these enormous needles to draw fluid off the spine. I was terribly frightened, although I was almost delusional with the fever. One of the earliest and sharpest memories I retain of that time was looking at her fingertips as I was squeezing the blood out of them and of the pain as they inserted those needles, and of the squeezing and squeezing, and I don't know if she was having a difficult time with me hurting her but I just remember focusing on those fingertips to distract myself from the pain and squeezing them and watching the blood flow out of them. I had three spinal taps in those first three days in the hospital. What was so terrible about the disease and those initial symptoms was the fever. It was sustained at about 107 for three or four or five days, and there was no bringing it down. It was simply a virus running its course. The doctors could try and comfort me with some medications. I was sleeping on a rubberized mattress filled with ice and water. I had never seen such a thing before. And they would change the water every so often because I would simply warm it up and it was time to get a cold-water bed again. Every time I shifted I could hear the crunch of the ice and the water sloshing underneath. I had endless days and nights of cold washcloths placed on my forehead and injections throughout the day. I don't know if they ever did any good, some of them were undoubtedly to ease pain. Others may have been experimental drugs, but there were a lot of needles and lot of injections every day.

At that point I had polio and spinal meningitis at the same time. As I understand, it was not uncommon for kids afflicted with the disease. It caused my neck to curve up in kind of a horseshoe shape and it was interesting when the doctors would come in and bring residents around to examine me. They all were fond of putting their hands under my neck and kind of measuring it, and after several days they were pleased because it was getting harder to squeeze two hands in under my neck the way it was bowed up over the mattress. That was one of the kind of crude but effective gauges they used to see if I was progressing at all and battling against the disease. Eventually, they were quite concerned. This disease affected the spine and was a great indicator of possible

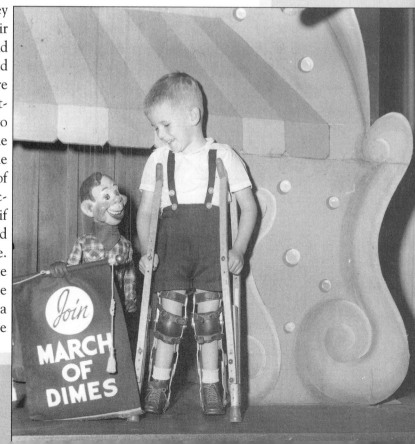

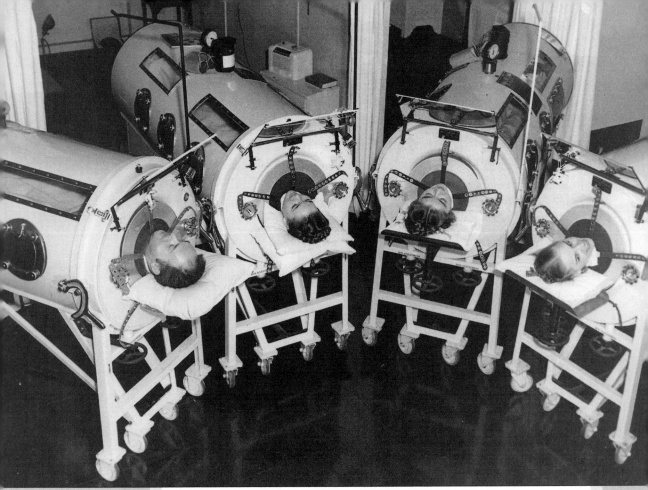

permanent paralysis, and they were pleased as the week went along and the fever started to break and my neck finally started to recover and return to normal.

The real frightening thing about being in the hospital was of course that the adults were so terrified, nervous, and upset, which carried directly to me. I didn't understand the disease. You're vaguely aware of it—they say the word polio, as a six-year-old it's something to dread, but it was really the reaction of the adults that I was playing off. Everyone who entered the room had to wear a mask and a gown because it was an isolated room. What struck me so much was the dramatic dealings of adults. I was laying there very sick with fever, in and out of consciousness and probably delusional at that time. The adults were very quiet, almost reverential, as they would come into the room. Doctors would murmur back and forth, they'd look at charts, they'd bring some specialists in. At times there'd be several people gathered at the foot of the bed and they would talk to one another in what to me was a foreign language. They spoke in hushed tones. They had a gravity about them that was dramatic to me. You constantly wondered what they're talking about, what conclusions they are reaching. They don't seem to reach any conclusions and if they do they are certainly not sharing them with you. It all added up to more fear and more uncertainty. It was a very terrifying thing to a young boy. Laying there in the bed wondering what had happened to me! A week before, I had been playing ball and was at the beach, romping around in the summertime. And now I was lying in this strange hospital, confined, with no one allowed to come in, with some disease that I didn't understand that was making me horribly sick, wondering how long I was going to be in there.

I wouldn't have much contact with any humans. The hospital workers were either so busy or not keen on coming into a room where there was such contagion. My parents were limited in their visitations. The doctors would come in, but only sporadically. So I was really isolated. Bed pans would pile up, dishes would pile up. I was not only very sick and afraid, but alone. I got to the point where I was too sick to get out of bed and no one was there to help me and I would soil my shorts there in bed. And one day my mother came in, outside of visiting hours, she simply couldn't stay away any longer. And I happened to be in the bathroom doing what moms did, which was washing out my underwear and soil. She saw a stack of bedpans and she saw a stack of dishes piled up, and saw me in there doing that and read the riot act to whoever was on duty at that time. It was at that time that she started to push hard to get me out of the hospital and to get me back home to rehabilitate there.

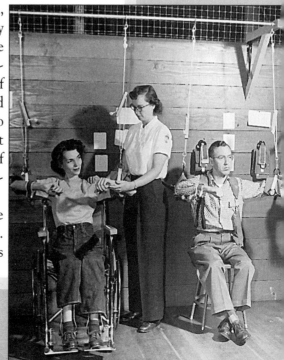

I remember at one point, my parents had come in and visited briefly, as they were allowed to do. And they said that they had positioned my sisters outside, down on the lawn outside the hospital, many floors below, and I saw them down there, both of them. They were waving to me, and so I actually got up there on the window ledge, and had my hands pressed up against it so they could see me very excited. This was toward the end of the week as the fever was breaking and I was feeling better.

Can you tell me a little bit about your rehabilitation?

Basically, the disease left me with weakened ankles and weakened lower legs. I had what they called a debutante swagger. I had a weakened hip and it caused me to kind of wiggle as I walked for a time after that. I was fitted with shoes that had a steel heel called a Thomas heel to shore up my ankles. I went to therapy once or twice a week for six months after I got out of the hospital, and I would have specialists who would examine how I was walking, correct my gait, give me exercises to work on to strengthen my ankles, strengthen my knees, and strengthen my lower legs. The doctors were very emphatic that I should try to get into athletics, especially ice hockey. Being in Detroit, all winter long the kids were skating. My dad was born in Canada and had played hockey all his life, so that was a natural. I actually had learned to skate when I was three years old, but with polio I had to learn to walk again, learn to literally put one foot in front of the other at age six. And then I finally got strong enough to begin running, and then got on an ice hockey team, and that seemed to really help. I made great progress because I pushed myself at the doctor's and my parent's urging to work on those lower limbs, to work on my ankles, to get stronger.

Tell me about getting the little sugar cubes with the Sabin vaccine.

I was at Thomas Edison School in Detroit at the time the sugar cube was introduced. The kids were told in advance that it was going to be quite an exciting thing. It was made into a very positive thing and of course everyone was encouraged to come and not miss that day. I had kind of a badge of honor because I had had polio. The adults put me in kind of a special category for that, and so when I went to get the sugar cube it was kind of a lark for me and I was happy to tell all my

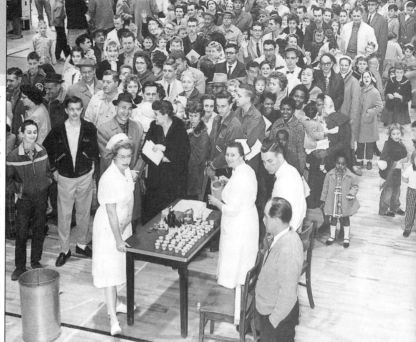

friends that I don't really need this, I have the natural immunity, I've gone through this, and I'm taking the sugar cube as precaution. You folks all need this sugar cube, I'm different, I'm special. So that experience was not nearly the important and grave moment that other parents undoubtedly made it out to be for their children. We lined up [outside] the gymnasium and we got inside and they handed us all a little Dixie cup and it had the sugar cube and I remember they were pink or blue. It was a rite of passage. You were supposed to feel something different. I don't know that any of us did, but the moment was really built up by the parents and teachers.

What did polio mean at that time in history?

It was the robber of childhood innocence, it was the robber of hope for a generation, several generations of children. There were diseases and scientists charted them, but none was more devastating, affected more children, was more deadly than polio. But polio left kids crippled and that was an image that this big, strong postwar country simply couldn't abide. We had children lining up in wheelchairs, in iron lungs, whose very vitality and everyone's hope for their future was allayed right at the most critical time in their childhoods. And that's why polio seemed like such a horrible scourge, far more so than any number of other diseases or accidents that, any way you want to measure it, were more deadly and were fatal. And the image of a child in an iron lung is about as tearful and wrenching as we could imagine at that time and any time certainly in this century.

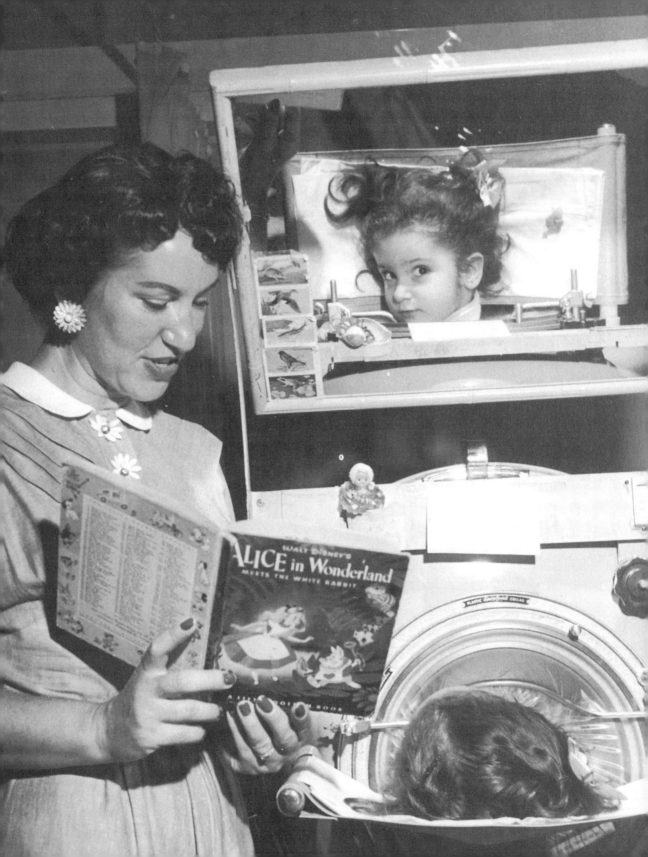

Arvid Schwartz

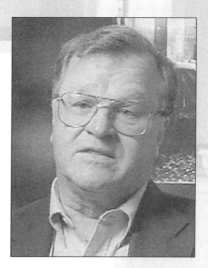

Arvid Schwartz was living on a farm in northern Minnesota when he came down with polio at age twelve. For over forty years he has walked with leg braces and crutches.

Tell me what happened when you first got sick; how you found out you had polio.

There were some early warning signs as we look back, or at least we think they were warning signs. I had taken a bad tumble with my bicycle and I was a pretty good bicycle rider. That was unlike me. And then I had some noticeable lameness in my legs. I had my chores to do on the farm and my father noticed that, but we didn't know it was polio. I realized something was wrong when I woke up on the third or fourth morning and had this flu. I stepped out of bed and fell flat to my face. I still had no thought of polio because that always happened to the neighbor kids or the other folks in town. I was twelve years old and I remember quite vividly my father carried me downstairs and put me on a daybed, and that's where I spent the next two to three days as the family debated what was wrong. Obviously, something was wrong but in 1952 in rural Minnesota you didn't go to the doctor the minute you ran a fever. You waited until you were sure something was wrong. So the most vivid moment was when I got out of bed and fell down. And I've never walked a step since that day without the aid of crutches and braces.

How did you find out that it was, in fact, polio?

I can remember that as though it happened five minutes ago. We had the doctor come out and he did not make a diagnosis right away. Everybody still thought I had some kind of flu. But it didn't go away and he came back, and then he mentioned the possibility of polio. It was the first time that awful word had been mentioned. He said we probably ought to go to the Twin Cities. He directed us to the University of Minnesota Hospital. I couldn't walk and my father had to get me into the backseat of our two-door car and prop me up with blankets and pillows. It was a very beautiful fall day, October 18. And I took a long look around the farm. I very much loved the farm, and I thought to myself, 'I better look around. I may not be back here for a while.' And that was more prophetic than I had hoped it might have turned out, for I didn't come back there for a long time.

My father had never driven to the Twin Cities in his life. He had only been there once before. We got to the University Hospital at the 5:00 rush hour. There I had my spinal and at 10:00 that night the hospital decided that I really needed to go to Sister Kenny because of the severity of the case. Sister Kenny did not have any room that day but they said, 'Bring him over, we'll find a place,' and that's exactly what they did. They found a very crowded place, and I can remember being on a gurney and my parents saying goodbye to me and being wheeled to a room amidst a lot of clatter of iron lungs, down to a room that was just wall-to-wall beds with people who had just been diagnosed. This was a contagion ward and that was where I spent the next eight days, totally laying on my back staring at the ceiling, crying a lot. I'd kind of relive my day at school to occupy myself those few days. I'd think, 'Well, it's 8:30, we'd be in school now, and its 9:30, we'd be having spelling or geography,' and I mentally went through the day just to keep track of the hours because I couldn't see a clock very well and I had to ask the nurse. And I cried a lot because I had no idea what was going to happen to me. I didn't really know if I had a fatal disease and if I was going to live or die. You have to visualize, I was one patient out of hundreds, and I didn't get any better or more special care then anyone else. I had to be catheterized, had to have enemas and it was a terribly distasteful experience.

Tell me about that moment of separation from your family.

At Sister Kenny they gave no information as to whether this was a one-week stay, or a one-month stay, and I remember my mother and father standing above me and taking my hand and saying goodbye. I

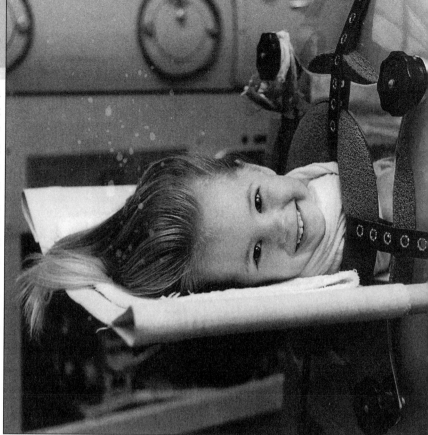

never have asked them what thoughts went through their mind. They were sent to a hotel about a block from Sister Kenny where most of the parents were sent. And I can imagine the agony they probably had that night and the whole week I was in contagion because I couldn't see them. They called the doctors, but again I was just one of many and they couldn't give me a specific diagnosis, of how much paralysis I was going to have, and so forth. We were just in a holding pattern to get me through that seven or eight days, to get the fever down and make sure nothing else happened.

What did you think about what was going on? What were your thoughts about polio?

I was too young, I suppose, to totally appreciate the consequences of what was going on, yet I was fully aware that my life probably was going to change from that moment. I can remember thinking about that in those early days, that all those dreams you have as a child kind of start to evaporate and vanish because things were totally different. There were three or four other people who had had polio earlier in our community and they had some residual effect, and so I was aware of what polio was. Two of those people were in wheelchairs and the other two had recovered almost completely. One of them walked with sticks or crutches, the other one unaided. So we thought about that, but you never ever thought that you would get polio. And [it turned out that] in the community where we lived, I was the last major polio victim. I

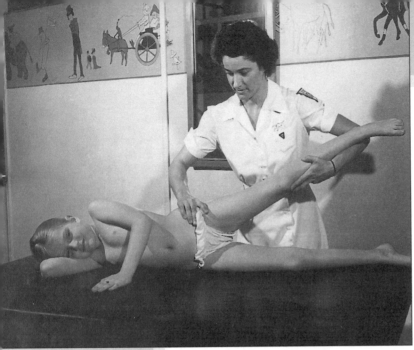

believe there was one other case after me, but that was a very, very mild case and it never left any effect on the person. And after 1953 polio started disappearing.

What happened after you were moved out of contagion?

I remember being put into this room where there were again a sea of beds. Not only against the wall, but beds down the middle where there was supposed to be an aisle. I wonder what the codes were about getting out in case of a fire because it was not going to happen. But I remember coming into that room and seeing all those strange faces, all young boys approximately my age, ten to fifteen. And I thought, 'I don't know anybody in here.' They put me up in the corner of the room and there was a young boy who came and introduced himself and his name was Dave Jenkins. He talked to me that first day and told me a little bit about polio and how it was going to change his life. That was the night my parents got to see me for the first time since we had parted seven or eight days earlier. Of course I was looking forward to that, but it was a very, very brief visit. Sister Kenny had very strict rules about visiting hours because of the volume of patients. I remember when they got there my mother was crying and my father's lip was trembling quite badly. I had never seen those things before as a kid. I guess I was the reassuring one. Perhaps I knew it would work out. My friend in the room said you've got to have special shoes and they were going to cost quite a bit of money. Quite a bit of money in those days was like $18 or $18.95. And of course I had never had a pair of shoes that cost that much, and I remember telling my parents that I needed these shoes and that they were really expensive. They said 'Don't worry about it, we'll figure that out.' Little did I know that I'd be there for seven or eight months and the cost of shoes would be just a footnote to the total bill, which ran into the thousands and thousands of dollars.

Were you helped by the March of Dimes?

Yes, we did not have health insurance. My father was a farmer and we certainly did not have the kind of money it would take to pay a bill of that magnitude. The March of Dimes helped us immensely. My father bought some of the accessories I needed like shoes, crutches, and braces. But I would say they paid in the high 90 percent. And my parents became quite active in that organization after that.

Can you tell me about your Sunday visits?

Sister Kenny had visiting hours on Sundays from 2:00 to 4:00 and that was the extent of when parents could see children. For eight months my parents made that trip from western Minnesota to the Twin Cities without fail, except for one Sunday when they got about halfway and had to turn around because of a snowstorm. You have to think back to the roads back then, plus my father had chores in the morning and chores in the evening when he got home. But they never missed a Sunday and I appreciated that because that was really my only face-to-face contact with my family.

I remember parents would sneak candy to their kids because Sister Kenny would absolutely prohibit anything that wasn't in their diet and so candy was just a complete no-no. Parents knew they weren't supposed to be doing it and the kids knew they weren't supposed to be getting it, but it was this great undercover operation that worked. And then it was up to us, after visiting hours were over, to hide that candy someplace. Now we didn't have a lot of places to hide things. It was a room with a lot of beds. There were a few little nightstands and we had knapsacks at the end of our beds that we hung over our bedposts, but that was the first place the nurses would always look. We would figure out how to get it under a mattress or between the mattress and the blanket, and of course some of that candy melted and we would have a mess. And every so often the nurses would have a raid after visiting hours. They would find all the candy and letters would go out to our parents from Sister Kenny reminding them that was inappropriate and they shouldn't be doing it. Of course parents at that time were fearful they were doing something wrong so there would be a two- to three-week period where there would be no candy. Then someone would get brave and the whole thing started all over again, and we'd work it up to where we had a pretty good supply and then another raid. And to this day I think the nurses knew what was going on all the time, but they kind of let us get by a little bit. I guess that's why at fifty-seven I still appreciate a candy bar.

Talk a little bit about the treatment.

The treatment for polio was hot packs, hot packs, and then some more hot packs. And then some stretching treatments. They would apply the hot packs to your lower extremities, your upper extremities, your back, your abdomen, wherever you had any paralysis. And they were hot, hot as you can stand. I remember them being too hot

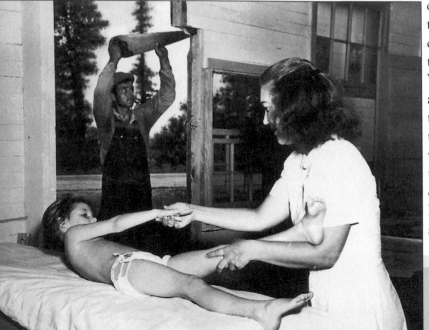

once in a while, and certain people in our room couldn't handle them and there would be screams. We would usually get two applications of those in the mornings and two in the afternoon and they would put them on leave them on for an hour and come back with some hotter ones, and it seemed like by the fourth one in the afternoon they just couldn't get them any hotter.

Some place during the day they would let you have a little time off and you would have stretching of a muscle. That was done with the therapists and then by a fellow by the name of Pat, who was a big guy. He must have been a wrestler at some time of his life and when it came to these stretching exercises those hurt because they were doing things to your body that the body didn't want to do any longer. The thing was, could you sit up and touch your head to your knee, could you get your leg straight, could you get your back straight? Try to do a sit-up. Try to push against

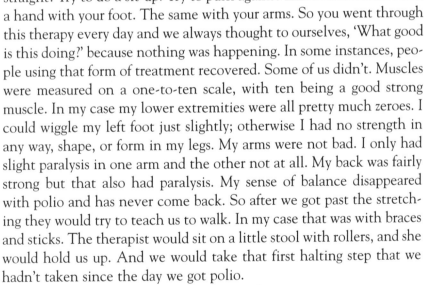

a hand with your foot. The same with your arms. So you went through this therapy every day and we always thought to ourselves, 'What good is this doing?' because nothing was happening. In some instances, people using that form of treatment recovered. Some of us didn't. Muscles were measured on a one-to-ten scale, with ten being a good strong muscle. In my case my lower extremities were all pretty much zeroes. I could wiggle my left foot just slightly; otherwise I had no strength in any way, shape, or form in my legs. My arms were not bad. I only had slight paralysis in one arm and the other not at all. My back was fairly strong but that also had paralysis. My sense of balance disappeared with polio and has never come back. So after we got past the stretching they would try to teach us to walk. In my case that was with braces and sticks. The therapist would sit on a little stool with rollers, and she would hold us up. And we would take that first halting step that we hadn't taken since the day we got polio.

Tell me about the first time you went home.

Christmas in 1952 they gave us polio patients a two-day pass to go home, those of us that were able. And they really did a superhuman effort to make most of us able to get home. We got out at 4:00 on Christmas Eve. That was the time we could leave, not a minute before.

And my parents took me home and I remember that vividly. We went into our little town, to the church where the Christmas program was going on. As we got there it had already started. I would have been participating in the program had I not gotten polio. And I remember parking outside the church and I could hear the sounds of 'Silent Night.' And that was pretty emotional. Still is.

We always had happy Christmases and this was a happy one also, but we didn't get any presents to speak of. It began to dawn on me that maybe there was a shortage of money. I remember that my brother had gotten a [model] car that I had built from a kit in the hospital and I thought, 'Gee, that's not much of a Christmas present.' That's all we had that Christmas, but I think my ability to be back at home was worth all that. It was an interesting experience. You can imagine that a house on the farm was about as handicapped inaccessible as it can get. We had no indoor plumbing or indoor running water, so we had to figure out how to make this all work. They had to carry me out to this little privy. The food that I had was all the things that I wanted, that I hadn't had, and of course it was absolutely the wrong thing to eat. We all came back to the hospital sick with the flu, diarrhea, and everything else, and parents were scared that they did something they shouldn't have, and we were scared. But I think the folks at Sister Kenny knew it was going to happen, and we were all nursed back to health in a few days.

Was there any kind of schooling for the children at Sister Kenny?
I was in the seventh grade at the time. I had gone to school through the middle of October until I became ill. But at Sister Kenny they made an attempt to have a school amongst all these kids, and they really did an excellent job. We went down to the cafeteria and had a little corner where we had our little schoolroom set up in the afternoon. There was a teacher, Mrs. Kagerryus, and perhaps five of us. I was able to be wheeled down in a chair, not a wheelchair, but a regular kitchen chair with casters under it. One kid came down in a bed with a respirator and we heard his respirator going. We had all our seventh grade classes, but it was all condensed into fifteen-minute versions so we were out of the cafeteria before the evening meal started.

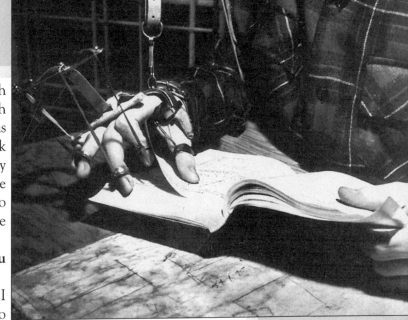

But that was my seventh grade. I guess I learned enough and I got a report card just as though I would have back home. The principal in my hometown got it, then made the decision to pass me on to the eighth grade. I think he was being kind.

Let's talk about when you finally got to go home.

About a month before I went home they moved me to what was then called Swedish Hospital in Minneapolis, and there I had my own room. The polio patients there were varying ages, both men and women, and we could do whatever we wanted. It was really open and free. Totally 180 degrees from Sister Kenny. We could go outside the hospital. We could take our wheelchairs and go up and down the streets. We could go to the corner store and buy something if we wanted to. I think it was a transition month. They didn't tell us this; I guess it was just part of the treatment, just to see how well we worked out. I remember one day they came and told me I could go home and, quite frankly, I hadn't even thought about going home. I resigned myself to thinking this was going to go on forever in the hospital, but they said, 'You're done. You can go home. You're as good as you're going to get. So call up your parents and tell them.' And I thought, 'Hmm, this is strange,' but obviously I called them right away. And I remember that next day, the 19th of June, 1953. I fretted that morning because I was sure something had gone wrong, that I just dreamt this, or my parents weren't going to get there, or they were going to come at the last minute and say, 'We've made a mistake and you really can't go home.' I [hardly] slept at all the night before until they actually walked in the room and we went home.

My bedroom was upstairs and we had no bedrooms downstairs. It was an old farmhouse with an old winding staircase and so my dad had

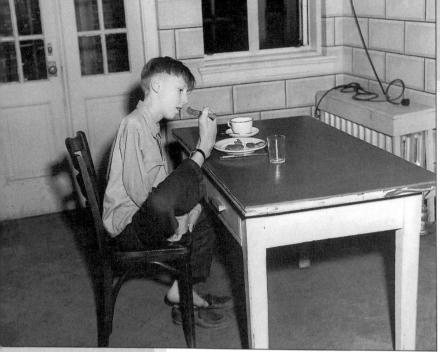

gone to the lumber yard and got a two-by-two and planed off the edges and nailed it to the wall, and that's how I made it upstairs. There weren't any aids, you just had to figure out how you were going to make this work and again it wasn't that my family wasn't interested in it. It just that at that time in the history of our country, when you were a cripple, as opposed to 'handicapped' or 'physically challenged,' you either made it or you didn't make it and it was kind of up to you to make it, with help from your family. There were no support groups, no programs, no classes you could go to. It doesn't make me a martyr. There were hundreds and hundreds of others who did the same thing and with far worse circumstances than I.

I spent the summer at home. In the fall I was going back to school, which was a one-room Christian school with one teacher. He was a very nice man and he came to visit me during the summer. I will remember him as long as I live. He just said, 'Of course, you're coming back to school. Why wouldn't you?' As though it wasn't worth talking about. So we didn't.

What happened when you went to school that fall?

The first day, I remember there was a coat room in the front and I remember having a moment of hesitancy as I walked inside. I was thinking, 'I am different.' I'm not the same as the rest of these kids, whom I knew and liked, and they liked me, but I was different. But I really couldn't turn back. My mother was with me and there wasn't anything to go back out for. You had to go to school, so I went to school. But I didn't participate in any of the things that kids that are thirteen or fourteen years old participated in. The teacher was very kind. We spent many noon hours and recesses playing checkers and Parcheesi and things like that. And even though he would have liked to get on the playground, because he was an athletic kind of guy, he spent his time with me, and saw to it that I was included in as much as I could. And if we got to a situation where I couldn't get up or down some steps he'd just pick me up and carry me. We didn't worry about who was going to be embarrassed, he or I, or the people around us. We just did it. And that's how it went for the eighth grade.

Then I had to go across the street to the big school, the public school, which has three and a half stories, and I thought, 'Now, how is this going to work?' I knew most of the kids, they had been in my confirmation class at church, but I didn't know all the teachers. And fortunately there was one other polio patient still in school, a young lady who was in a wheelchair, so I knew they had to have some idea how they were going to deal with this. We had two minutes between bells and classes, and I was expected to get from the bottom floor to the top floor in the same two minutes as everybody else. Nobody ever even asked me if it would take longer. They just assumed I was going to get there, as was the young lady in the wheelchair. Four guys grabbed her wheelchair and up the stairs she went. That's the way it was. Someone would carry my books for me. That was the only consolation that was given to me. So you just figured out how to do it. You knew what you were doing wasn't looking real good, and your methods perhaps weren't real graceful, but you had to do it. You had to get to where you had to get to, whether it was in school or whatever. And so I went through four years of high school, had a wonderful time and went to a school with wonderful kids and wonderful teachers and had just warm, warm experiences in spite of not having any kind of special privilege given to me.

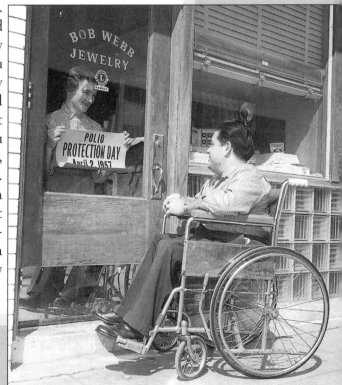

You had been athletic prior to getting polio. How did you stay involved in sports in school?

It really bothered me in the early stages. I wanted to be involved. As teenagers we didn't want to be left out. But the coach, a rough, gruff old guy, said, 'Well, why don't you be the student manager of these sports teams?' And I suddenly became part of the group. I rode the players' bus, I was friends with the players and the cheerleaders. But dating. I mean, I was a cripple. Who was going to go out with a cripple? As harsh as it sounds today, that is what you were called. And all those things were sort of traumatic. I went through a lot of fear, thinking, 'When I'm out of high school my world will kind of come to an end.' I kind of had visions that I would spend the rest of my life at home, which I did not want to do. I guess the biggest fear I had was that I would never marry. I was sure that I could be married and I could have a family, and I could be a father and a good husband and all of those things. But you know, I had to find someone else that might be interested in that same scenario, and I did. And she's been my best friend, my partner for thirty-five years. So it all worked out.

Tell me what went through your mind when the vaccine came out?

You know, when the Salk vaccine was announced, even in its preliminary stage, I was still in Sister Kenny. And I guess the thought that I had, and I think most of us had in the hospital, was it didn't come soon enough for us. But what is even more vivid is that we just missed it by a minute. Had I not gotten polio until five months later, maybe I wouldn't have gotten it. Although you have to look at that with a certain amount of philosophy too, because in rural Minnesota I doubt there was any Salk vaccine in 1953. So, it's just one of those things that happened, it was supposed to happen, and I guess I rejoiced, as most parents did, as we grew up in the 1960s and 1970s, that our kids didn't have to worry about polio.

What has having the disease meant to your life?

Well, in every cloud they say there is always a silver lining. And you just have to look for it. With polio, like any other disease that destroys the body either physically or even mentally, you have to figure out where's the good in this? And that's perhaps the most difficult part. But, as I think back on my forty-some years since I've had polio, I really can't think of anything that was bad because I had polio, after you got by the moment. It has certainly taught me to be a person with a much bigger heart than I might have had had I not had polio. Sure, I'd like to walk. You know I never carried my bride across the threshold and I was too big for her to carry me, so that didn't happen. I never carried my child. I

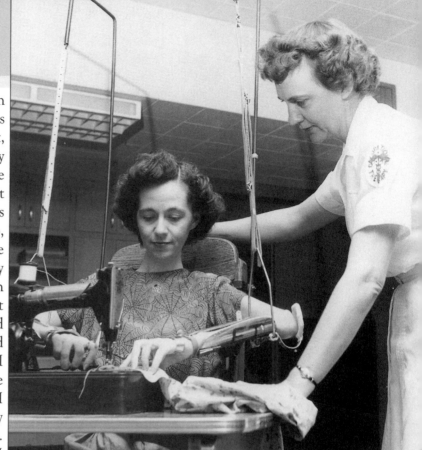

never carried a bag of groceries in my life. But I've had a lot of other experiences that other folks haven't had, and so I don't fret about not being able to walk, or not being able to ride a bike, even though that may be kind of interesting again. I have two philosophies that I kind of use: one of them is that life is a deck of cards. You either play them or you throw them in. I think that playing them is better than throwing them in. And the second one is you waste a lot of valuable time sitting around trying to figure out what might have been. You take what you have, and you go with it. And that's what I've done all my life. And as I've said to other people who've asked me this, I simply say, 'To God alone be the glory.'

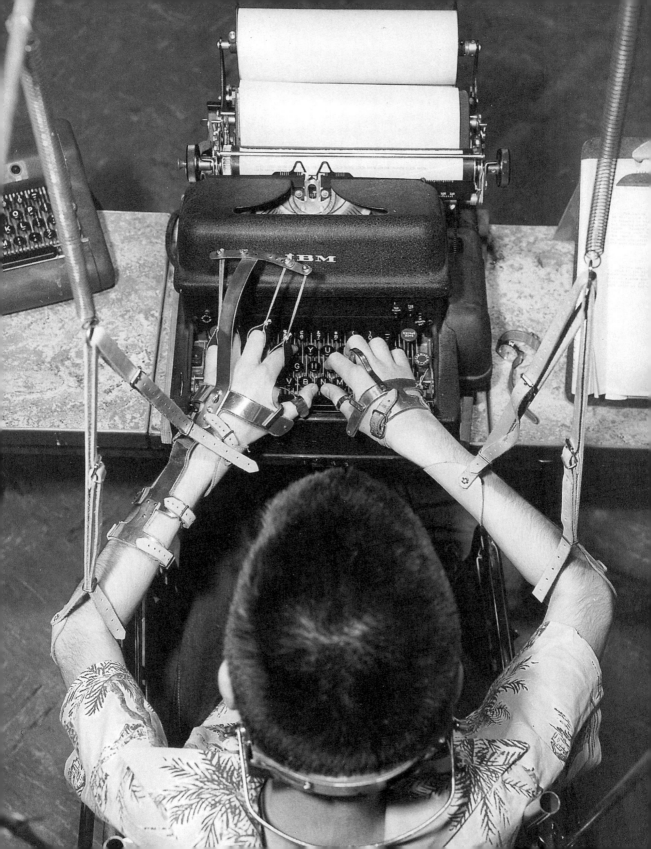

David Kangas

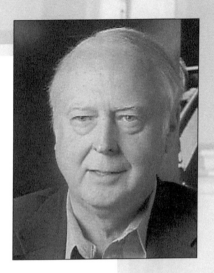

David Kangas was fifteen years old when he was playing in a marching band at a polio benefit parade in Hibbing, Minnesota. He noticed that his legs were weakening and he dropped out of line at the march. He was in the first stages of polio that would leave him without the ability to use his legs again.

Tell me what you knew about polio before you got it.

I knew virtually nothing. I knew that parents and other people would talk about it and be very concerned about it. [My parents] were always warning me during the polio season not to go to the beaches and we were always supposed to wash the fruit and things of that sort.

What happened when you first got polio?

The first indication that I knew something was wrong was during physical education during the school day. I was fifteen. We were all playing touch football and I noticed my right leg was just sort of weak and would buckle under me. There wasn't any pain. It was just a weakness. It wasn't until that evening that I became ill. I was in Hibbing, marching in the polio benefit parade with the high school band. I played cornet. And as I marched the weakness in my legs became more pronounced. I finally had to drop out of the march and sit on the curb because I couldn't go any further.

After the parade was completed, I found my way back to the school bus. We went out to the stockcar racetrack. The stockcar races were actually the event that generated the income for the benefit. And the band had been invited to watch the races, but I was feeling more and more sick so I stayed in the bus, I just lay down on the bus seat, and after a while the band director came back to see how I was and he noticed how bad I was feeling and decided to find a car and drove me the thirty miles back home. When I got home my parents of course were very concerned and they saw that I was becoming more and more weak and that I could hardly walk any longer. They actually put me in a bathtub; they thought that could relax my muscles. The doctor came and said it may be polio. He said we should drive back to Hibbing Hospital. It was about midnight when we got there. I didn't know what was happening. I'd never been in a hospital before. I walked into the hospital, walked down the hall to my room and that was the last time I walked ever again.

What was the course of events in the hospital?

The next day they did a spinal tap to confirm the polio diagnosis. My muscles eventually became weak to the point that they felt it was better if I was placed in an iron lung. It looked ominous. They open one end and slide the stretcher-type thing into the tank and then closed it. From then on you're taken care of by a nurse putting her hands through the arm holes in the side of the iron lung. I wasn't struggling to breathe like I was before. I was in a room with another boy my age, and he was in an iron lung also. And I remember that he seemed to be suffering from the pain a lot more than I was, for some reason, and he would cry out very loudly all night long. The nurses would come and try and comfort him. The nurses did a tremendous job.

Was there a response from your school about your getting polio?

It was quite an event in that I was the only student in the school that had polio and of course the story of my marching in the polio benefit parade in Hibbing resulted in sort of a newsworthy thing, that was written up in the newspapers. And a picture of me in the iron lung appeared in the papers. There was a fellow, Ed Monacelli, from a neighboring town who read the story and was so taken with it that he asked the nurses at the hospital what an iron lung would cost and found out it was about $2,600. That was the amount of money he'd saved up for a new car, and he said, 'Well, tell the sisters at the hospital to order an iron lung for David or for anyone else who needed it. I'd rather use the money that way.'

What happened after that week?

It was a great relief to get out of the iron lung and to be able to breathe normally on my own. After that it was the period of having to endure the hot packs, the Kenny treatments, and the exercises with the physical therapist. The therapist would sometimes get right up on the table and put your leg on their shoulder and pull with their hands on your knee to straighten out your leg and stretch the muscles. It was painful and you yelled a lot, but they said, 'We need to do this so you won't tighten up.'

Jim and Joanne were the physical therapists at Hibbing Hospital and they had quite a workload. Jim had just come out of physical therapy school and was hit with this epidemic of polio persons all needing a lot of therapy. I remember Jim and Joanne working ten- to twelve-hour days with the patient load that they had. Jim told me later, 'Sometimes I really didn't know what I was doing. This was my first polio epidemic and I had to handle all these patients.' They both worked very hard and helped me a lot.

I was looking forward to going home for Thanksgiving, and of course in my mind it was a matter of walking out of the hospital and going home. They did let me visit at home for Thanksgiving but it meant a ride in an ambulance. I came back after Thanksgiving and stayed until Christmas. Came home for Christmas, then went back to Hibbing, and it was during January and February when we began thinking about transferring down to Sheltering Arms Hospital in Minneapolis. We were told that they had more intensive treatment, so in March we made the trip down to the city and I entered the hospital there. They told me

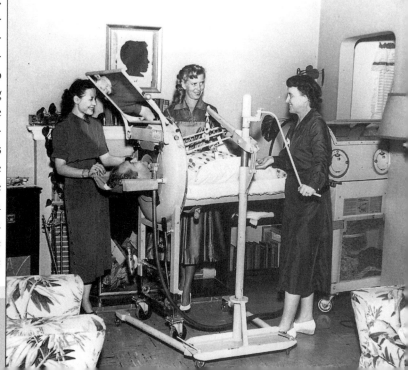

they had some whirlpool baths, but when we got to the hospital we said, 'Show me where your whirlpool baths are.' We were taken to a room where there were several ordinary bathtubs. And I said, 'These aren't whirlpool baths,' and I always remember the person who took me there said, 'The only whirl you'll get here is watching the water go down the drain.' We found out later that, actually, the benefit of Sheltering Arms was to really continue your therapy for range-of-motion and to get you start to thinking about what your life would be as a person with a disability.

When did you realize that you wouldn't get well?

Probably the beginning of that summer, because I met so many more patients at Sheltering Arms who had polio long before me, and I began to see that you had to deal with what muscles had been left to you and to do the best you could. I realized I would not walk again and I would need to do the best I could with a wheelchair and crutches or braces. So I decided that it wouldn't do me much good to stay there any longer and I really wanted to go home. I had been in the hospital for nine or ten months, so I asked the doctor to discharge me and he did.

How did you feel?

I had a great feeling of loss. I had looked forward to the previous school year. I was active at sports and band and all the school activities, and that didn't seem to be possible any longer. That summer, the

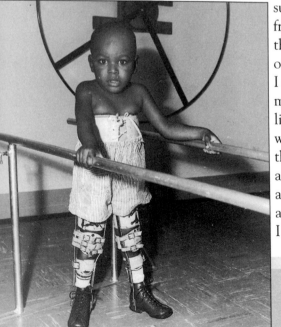

summer of 1953, I got together with some of my friends and they were looking forward to working for the city—cutting the grass in the park and doing other odd jobs—and I tried to figure out something I could do. So we went down and I talked to the foreman and said, 'You usually hire teenage boys, and I'd like to work this summer also.' Well, I was in a wheelchair, of course, and he said, 'Oh, what do you think you can do?' I said, 'Well, you paint the curbs and the lines for the parking spaces every summer, and I could certainly do that.' And he said, 'Give it a try.' And he gave me a chance, and a paint bucket. I hooked the paint can onto the handle of my wheel-

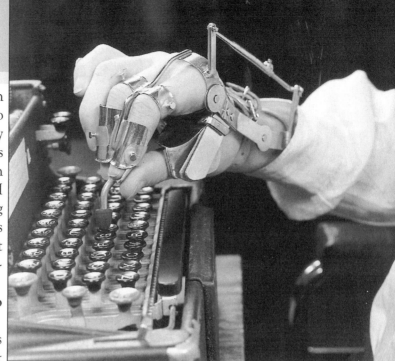

chair, and I would move down the line. And when I needed to move across I always had my friend grab the paint. He was always bringing the paint can one step ahead of me so that I wouldn't have to be reaching back for it all the time. It was sort of a teamwork deal and it worked well. It was a great feeling to be able to work.

Tell me about going back to school that fall.

The school, of course, was not wheelchair accessible. It was a two-story school and there were steps on the outside to get in, and then steps up to the second floor. There were no elevators—well, there was a freight elevator, which didn't work very well for me. So, what I needed to do was to arrange to have my friends grab the wheelchair and carry me up and down the steps to my classes, and this is how I got back into the school routine. I was the president of my class, although I missed most of the sophomore year. When I got back to school for the junior year, I took part in most of the activities of the class president. I would have been on the basketball team that year and I was still interested in how the team was doing. But I was still not comfortable with crowds and a lot of people looking at me. So I arranged to be brought to the projection booth that was part of the auditorium and I thought maybe I could be in there and watch the game. Well, the word got around that I was attending the game and that I was up in the projection booth, and so everybody was looking up to the booth to see if they could see me and it was a little bit uncomfortable. But after the game, when I came down and was brought to the doors of the school, a lot of people came up and shook my hand and told me how glad they were to see me and I began to see that these people were my friends and it was okay.

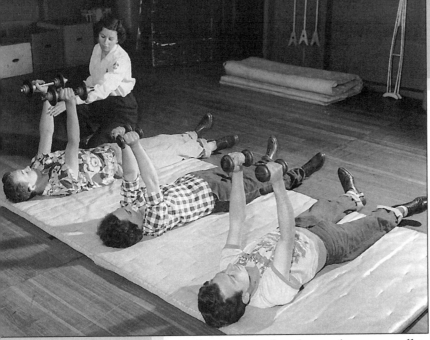

Can you tell me about your experiences at University of Minnesota?

I enrolled at the university not really checking things out, in terms of accessibility, and I found out, to my surprise, that there were hardly any buildings that were accessible with a wheelchair. So it was a matter of many times trying to pull together a crew of students who were walking by and ask, 'I need to get to the second floor of this building for my class, could you help me?' Sometimes they were very generous in doing so, but other times they were themselves rushing to another class and would say, 'I really can't, I need to get to this class' or 'I have a bad back, I can't really do this.' Maybe they did, maybe they didn't, and you just tried to get enough people together to give you a boost.

What is the enduring effect of polio on your life?

Well, I suppose the enduring thing is that I have learned that you can do a lot of things if you are persistent, work hard, figure out things. There is more than one way to do something and a lot of ways to solve a particular problem. It's a matter of solving one problem after another. I think it's made me more tolerant of people, with just a more empathetic view on life probably.

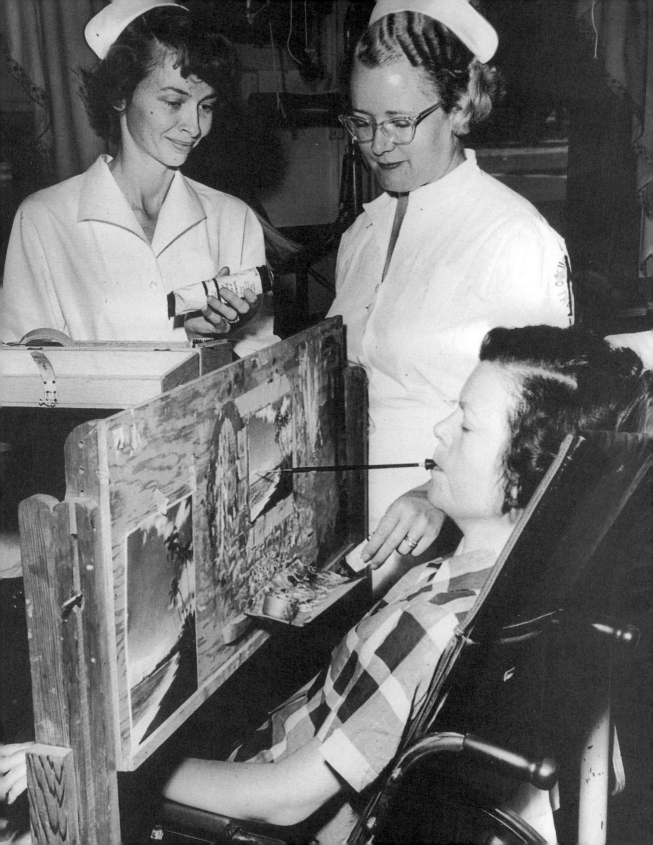

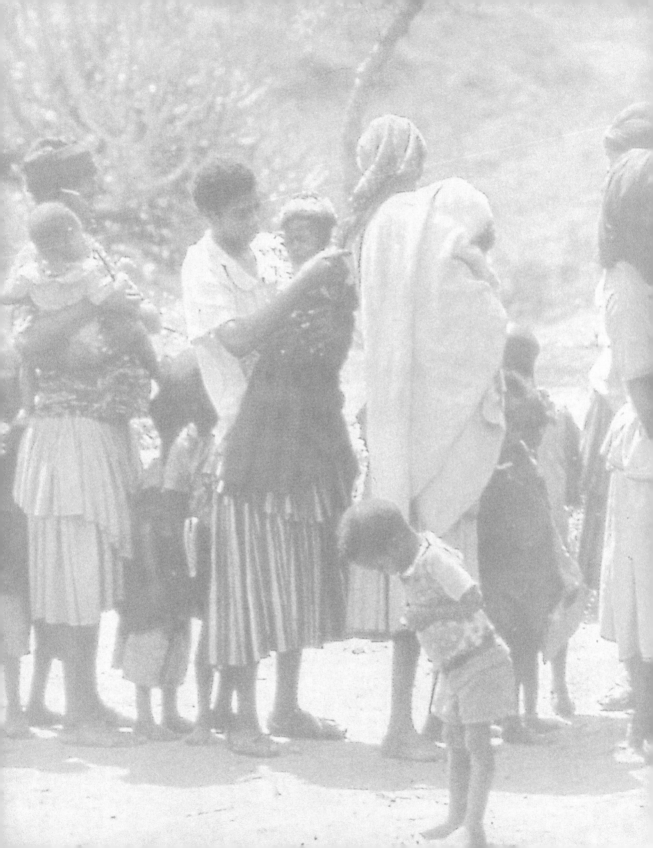

Afterword
Global Safety, Global Threats

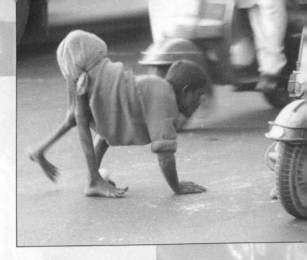

Today, the crippler poliomyelitis has been eradicated throughout the Western hemisphere. The last documented case in the Americas of paralytic polio caused by a wild virus was reported in Peru in 1991. A very small number of people, generally fewer than ten per year, are injured by vaccine-associated poliomyelitis, but the threat of polio epidemics has all but vanished. In less than fifty years, we have forgotten what it was like to live with the constant fear of polio. For most people, polio is not something they think about at all.

Unfortunately, that is not true in all parts of the world. Polio remains endemic in sub-Saharan Africa, Central Asia, South Asia, and scattered areas of the Western Pacific, the Eastern Mediterranean basin, and Europe. As recently as 1992, carriers of wild polio virus from the Indian subcontinent seeded outbreaks in Jordan, Malaysia, and the Netherlands, which in turn became the source of a series of infections in a small community in Canada that had refused vaccination for religious reasons. More recently, epidemics have broken out in Sudan in 1993, in Pakistan and Zaire in 1995, and in Albania in 1996.

Since polio strikes only humans and has no natural home outside the human body, current efforts are turned toward eliminating the disease entirely. In 1985, thirty years after the licensing of the Salk killed-virus injected vaccine and twenty-five years after the introduction of the Sabin live-virus oral vaccine, Rotary International, the service organization, made the eradication of polio the major activity of its 1.2 million members. At that time, over forty thousand cases of polio per year were still being reported worldwide, and many public health officials doubted that a private organization, with little experience in

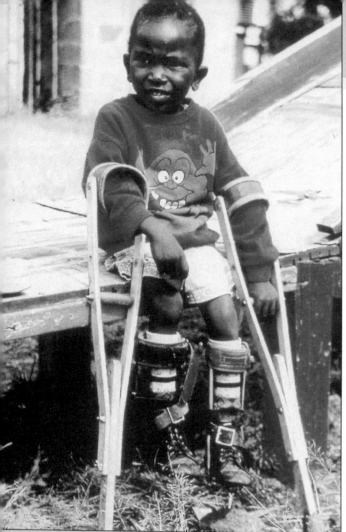

either health care programs or international activities, would have any success in such a massive enterprise. Happily, the skeptics were wrong. The combination of the international fundraising ability and a global network of local volunteers has enabled Rotary to function on an international scale much as the March of Dimes did in the United States. Money raised by Rotarians around the world funds the purchase of the vaccine and of the equipment needed to distribute it, while local Rotary clubs mobilize public support and provide volunteer workers, without whom it would be difficult if not impossible to run vaccination clinics.

The mission to eliminate polio gained further support in 1988, when the World Health Organization set the goal of global eradication by the year 2000. In that year, there were over thirty-five thousand cases reported worldwide. By 1997, the annual toll had dropped to approximately thirty-five hundred, a stunning reduction but still far short of total eradication. Epidemiologists estimate that reported cases represent at best 10 percent of the actual incidence of infection, and it is well-known that people who show no signs of polio may still spread the virus to more vulnerable contacts. Given the ease of travel to and from even remote parts of the world, we cannot take any comfort in our distance from the centers of disease. As long as polio is endemic in Turkistan, sub-Saharan Africa, India, or anywhere else on earth, no person anywhere is completely safe. Until every child is vaccinated—and every area of the globe declared free of polio—vaccination programs will have to continue everywhere.

It takes a tremendous effort to vaccinate every child on earth, and it costs a great deal of money. The coordinated efforts of Rotary International, the World Health Organization, UNICEF (United Nations International Children's Emergency Fund), the United States Centers for Disease Control, and other health organizations, working with the cooperation of national governments, has led to programs of National Immunization Days that are on an even larger scale than the efforts in the United States to first test and then distribute the Salk and Sabin vaccines. In 1996, over 52 million children in sub-Saharan Africa were immunized during the "Kick Polio Out of Africa" campaign. Worldwide, four hundred million children, almost two-thirds of the global population of children under five, received vaccinations that year. On a single day in January, 1997, 127 million children were immunized in India. Separate programs send supplies, health workers, and volunteers to China, Laos, Myanmar, and Vietnam, and to under-served countries of the Mediterranean, Caucasus, and Central Asian Republics.

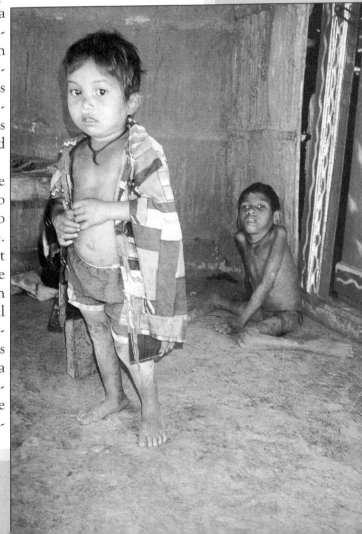

These efforts have led to a massive drop in the size and frequency of polio outbreaks, but it is still too early to celebrate the end of the disease. Impoverished regions often cannot afford either vaccine supplies or the refrigeration units needed to maintain vaccine potency. Wars and regional conflicts destroy the health care infrastructure; while reporters like to focus on the poignant moment when a cease-fire is declared to allow immunization, it is far more often the case that wars interrupt vaccination pro-

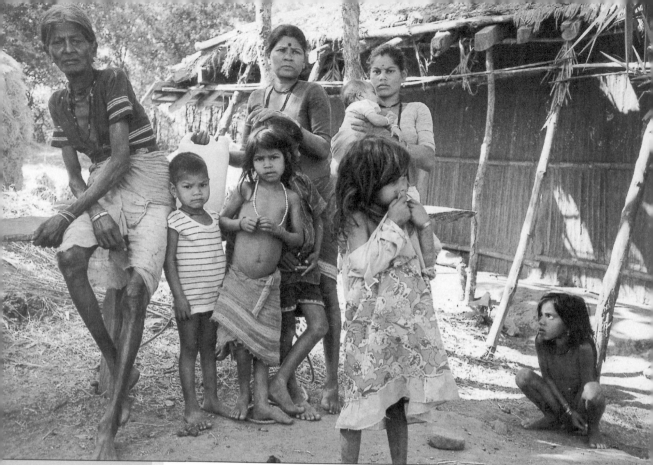

grams, leaving children unprotected at a time when malnutrition, stress, breakdowns in sanitary systems, and forced migrations make them particularly vulnerable to epidemic disease. National Immunization Days cannot be repeated soon enough to protect the youngest babies from polio, while the general rise in immunization and sanitation keeps them from the early exposure that had once limited injury among populations in undeveloped areas. In some regions, even aggressive vaccination efforts have failed to eliminate polio; despite massive vaccination programs, polio is still endemic in India, where there are over one thousand cases identified each year.

To conquer polio, many believe, we must copy the successful eradication of smallpox, which was achieved through a massive, simultaneous, global program of vaccination. According to the World Health Organization, it will cost an estimated $800 million to eradicate polio. If that happens, however, the economic benefits will be even greater.

Because polio is not carried by animals, a global vaccination program would effectively eliminate the virus—and with it, eliminate the need to vaccinate future generations. Health officials estimate that the savings from polio eradication would equal $230 million dollars every year, if routine immunization could be abandoned in the United States, as it has been for smallpox. Globally, $1.5 billion is spent every year on polio immunization—money that could be devoted to other health services if vaccination were no longer necessary.

The global eradication of polio will require more than worldwide vaccination, however. Before anyone can abandon vaccination, it will also be necessary to have a worldwide surveillance system to make sure that no pockets of infection persist. Without surveillance, there is the lingering possibility that the wild virus will continue to circulate in isolated areas, which could later become the source of new epidemics; if vaccination programs are halted prematurely, a new generation of children will be vulnerable to the disease. A worldwide surveillance program would provide early warning of other emerging viruses as well as of late outbreaks of polio. But it remains to be seen if governments and international agencies will be able to muster the same support for the extremely low-profile work of monitoring health trends, which they have been able to raise for the battle against the very visible threat of crippling poliomyelitis.

As we approach the new millennium, it is possible but not at all certain that goal of eradication by the year 2000 will be met. Until we have achieved global immunization against polio, and have matched that feat with the

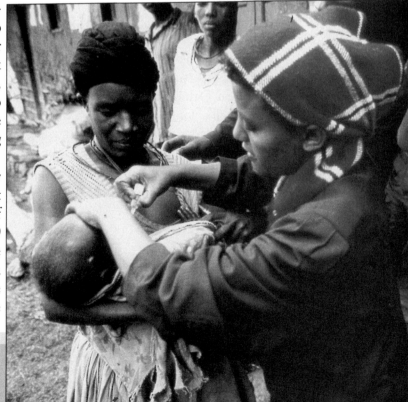

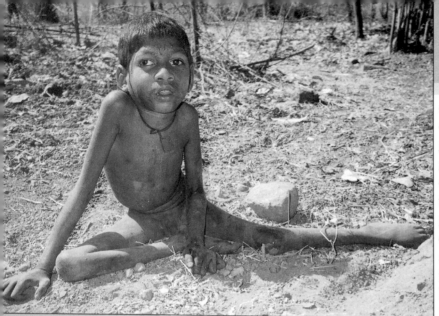

even more difficult but equally important goal of global surveillance, the greatest danger is complacency. Living without the fear of polio can be a dangerous bliss. Many children in the United States still do not receive the full complement of childhood vaccinations until they are legally required to do so to enter school. In 1991, only 53 percent of American children under four had received their full polio immunization, and vaccination rates in inner city areas of New York and Houston were lower than those in Cairo, Bangkok, or Bombay. Although there have been no cases of naturally-occurring polio in the United States since 1979, it is still possible that an epidemic could spread within a young and vulnerable population of unvaccinated children.

Polio occupies a unique place in the annals of medicine as a disease that was identified and conquered within a century. As the country that bore the brunt of the first epidemics and worked the hardest to find a protective vaccine, the United States has always looked on the conquest of polio as a story of national triumph, part of the saga of America. Now it is time to look beyond nationality, to recognize this saga to its conclusion. With a great deal of effort and a measure of luck, we may achieve global eradication of this dread disease. It is a goal we must pursue, for the world has become much too small for polio.

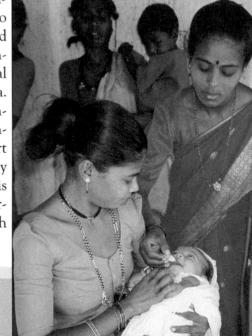

Catalog of Archival Photographs

All images are courtesy of the March of Dimes Birth Defects Foundation unless otherwise noted.

p. 3: This posed photograph conveys the "ray of hope" provided by the March of Dimes in its fights against polio.

Chapter 1

p. 18–19 background: A polio ward during the 1916 epidemic. (Courtesy of the Library of Congress)

p. 19: A 1918 image of a physician taking the blood from a man as the doctor conducted his research to develop a serum to combat polio. (Courtesy of Corbis–Bettmann)

p. 20: In the early part of the century, any public health menace would be handled in the same way: clean the streets in the hope that less dirt would mean less disease. While this was a preventative for many diseases, this would not be the prescription for polio. (Courtesy of the Library of Congress)

p. 21: During the 1916 epidemic, thousands of New Yorkers fled the city in order to avoid polio. (Courtesy of Corbis–Bettmann)

p. 23: In the 1916 epidemic, children and families were quarantined when a child contracted polio. For many, this meant hours spent indoors during the heat of the summer in the tenement housing of New York City. (Courtesy of Corbis–Bettmann)

p. 24: City emergency hospital.

p. 26: Care in the iron lung is constant—a patient needed to be cleaned, fed, and suctioned. When there was time, overworked nurses might be able to converse with the patients.

p. 28: The primary treatment for polio was hotpacking. This process entailed placing wool blankets in steaming hot water, wringing them out, and wrapping a patient's body with them. This small child is entirely enclosed in these hotpacks.

p. 29: The iron lung and the leg braces were the principal pieces of equipment associated with the polio epidemics.

p. 31: Specially built ambulances transported iron lung patients from local hospitals to regional respiration centers sponsored by the March of Dimes.

p. 32: In 1940 Australian physical therapist Sister Elizabeth Kenny brought new rehabilitation techniques to the U.S. Using hot packs and extensive muscle reeducation, Sister Kenny's techniques revolutionized the care of polio patients throughout America, aiding their recovery.(Courtesy of Corbis–Bettmann)

p. 33: Learning to take a stroll outside and ride a bike again after polio meant a liberation from the typical hospital routine.

p. 36: Helping a child to stand up again for the first time was a moment of achievement for both the physical therapist/nurse and the young patient.

p. 37: This child turns the page of his book by use of an automatic page-turner attached to his chin.

p. 38: A young mother sees her newborn for the first time, having delivered the infant while she was confined to the iron lung.

p. 40: A young boy is tested for polio in rural America by a visiting nurse.

p. 41: The ride to the hospital with a

feverish polio child was frequently one of the most difficult trips ever taken by a family.

p. 43: This early iron lung would have been used in the 1930s and early 1940s.

Chapter 2

pp. 44–45 background: FDR picnics with other polios and their friends and families at Warm Springs.

p. 45: Basil O'Connor, President of the March of Dimes (right) and Nicholas Schenck, Chairman of the Motion Pictures March of Dimes (left) present FDR with a million dollar check at the White House raised by movie theaters nationwide in the fight against polio in 1943.

p. 46: Because FDR could not walk and therefore a sense of power could not be conveyed by a towering stature or bustling movement, he developed a remarkable physical presence by a robust grin and characteristic jaunty pose with his cigarette holder. (Courtesy of the FDR Library)

p. 47: Eleanor and Franklin in a private moment. (Courtesy of the FDR Library)

p. 48: Outside of the swimming pool at Warm Springs, Georgia, Franklin Delano Roosevelt lunches with other polio patients during the warm water therapy. (Courtesy of the FDR Library)

p. 49: FDR seemed to walk, but in fact he had deftly learned to use his upper body strength to gracefully haul his paralyzed legs, that were locked straight in leg braces. (Courtesy of the FDR Library)

p. 50: Donald Anderson, poster boy for the 1946 NFIP campaign, lays a wreath at Franklin Roosevelt's grave. His comment was, "He was like me, he had infantile paralysis."

p. 52: When iron lungs were not available, an emergency oxygen tent might suffice for a breathing impaired patient, but usually an iron lung would have to be found as the paralysis continued.

p. 53: This early iron lung would have been used in the 1930s and 1940s.

p. 54: This polio patient is learning to walk down stairs again, managing both crutches and leg braces.

p. 55: Besides learning to walk again, occupational therapists helped small children play games and manipulate the sometimes small pieces needed to play them.

p. 56: Solarium at Warm Springs.

p. 57: A birthday party in honor of Franklin Roosevelt at Warm Springs attended by those who benefited from his founding of the rehabilitation center.

p. 58: A postage stamp issued honoring FDR which is indicative of his first love—not the White House, but the "Little White House" at Warm Springs.

p. 59: In spite of the fact that hundreds, sometimes thousands, of people saw FDR being helped or carried from his car or down an aisle, the subject of his disability was rarely discussed. (Courtesy of the FDR Library)

p. 60: Always at home at Warm Springs, FDR lounges in his bathing suit near the pool. Notice his legs withered by polio and the size of his developed torso that carried his weight when needed. (Courtesy of the FDR Library)

pp. 61 and 62: The only two known photographs of FDR in his wheelchair. No public photographs were ever allowed to be taken of FDR's reliance on a wheelchair despite the fact that he never walked and used a wheelchair every day of his life after the onset of polio at age thirty-nine. The two photographs were held in his private collection. (Courtesy of the FDR Library)

p. 63: One of FDR's favorite pastimes at Warm Springs was picnics with other polios and their friends and families.

p. 64: President Roosevelt dines with polio patients at Warm Springs.

p. 65: Alone, FDR was contemplative and unconcerned that his leg braces were captured by this photographer.

Chapter 3

pp. 66–67 background: March of Dimes fundraising rally.

p. 67: Basil O'Connor, President of the National Foundation for Infantile Paralysis and the March of Dimes, counts some of the many dimes that came in to help the fight against polio.

p. 68: Basil O'Connor, President, National Foundation for Infantile Paralysis and the March of Dimes.

p. 69: Emergency fundraising drives were held during summer epidemics using all available imagery to demonstrate the great need.

p. 70: Eddie Cantor, the famous radio personality who coined the phrase "March of Dimes," in a promotion for the National Foundation for Infantile Paralysis.

p. 71: Baseball great Willie Mays went to bat for the March of Dimes at the Polo Grounds in 1954.

p. 72 top: A young Frank Sinatra collects for the March of Dimes.

p. 72 bottom: Zsa Zsa Gabor pitches for the fight against infantile paralysis.

p. 73: March of Dimes campaigns were not just limited to the Mothers' March, the movie theaters, or the dime cards; here, solicitation takes place as city busses go by.

p. 74: Fundraising rallies and dance marathons for polio were part of a strategy for keeping public commitment high.

p. 75: Fear, pity, hope, and the notion that "this could be my child" were the emotions played upon by the March of Dimes fundraising campaigns.

p. 76: Carol Boyer, poster child.

p. 78: A sea of beds filled with children was housed in the gymnasium of a church to accommodate the onslaught of polio patients.

p. 79: Every aspect of living—feeding, bathing, and body eliminations—must be taken care of for the iron lung patient.

p. 80: President Dwight Eisenhower (foreground) with poster child and Basil O'Connor, President of the March of Dimes (background).

p. 82: Fundraising for the March of Dimes.

p. 83: Eleanor Roosevelt with her granddaughter Nina and her grandson Haven. Nina and Haven both contracted polio in the 1952 epidemic, but with no lasting effects.

p. 84: Poster child at fundraising rally in New York City.

p. 86: This ward at Rancho Los Amigos in Hondo, CA in 1952 is filled with iron lungs and rocking beds during America's largest epidemic. (Courtesy of Rancho Los Amigos)

p. 87: Iron lungs and hot packing machines being rushed from New York to Des Moines, Iowa, during the 1946 epidemic.

p. 88: When a patient was in the iron lung and needed bathing or bedding changed, a pressure dome would be closed over the head to allow assisted respiration to continue.

p. 89: While still needing respiration assistance, many children were able to keep up with the schooling they were missing during their long rehabilitation.

p. 90: A polio patient in arm slings learns to write and manage a cup again.

p. 91: Danny Kaye (left) and Bing Crosby (right) pose with a March of Dimes poster child for a fundraising campaign.

p. 92: Howdy Doody and the March of Dimes Poster Child made a powerful pitch to America's middle class in the early days of television.

p. 93: Mothers during the Mothers'

March pose with a poster child to advertise the local campaign.

p. 94: A radiothon for polio is the precursor to today's telethons for fighting disease.

p. 95: Dr. Albert Sabin in his lab in Cincinnati, Ohio.

p. 97: March of Dimes promotion at a movie house in New York City.

Chapter 4

pp. 98–99 background: An iron lung ward.

p. 99: Sometimes the hardest hit were adults. Here, a father comes home from the hospital still on a respirator. The children may have had the polio virus but without any symptoms and transmitted that virus to their father who then developed a severe paralytic form of the disease.

p. 100: A mother and child wait outside a tent hospital.

p. 101: An acute phase isolation unit, where patients were kept until they were no longer considered infectious.

p. 102: After surgery for polio, patients were frequently put in full body casts to straighten their spines for up to a year. Cutting a child out of a cast could sometimes be treacherous.

p. 103: Polio patients spent hours relearning the simple tasks that once had come to them without a thought.

p. 104: In segregated wards in the South, these black children received respiratory care. For long term care, the only place where black children could be accommodated was at the Infantile Paralysis Center at Tuskegee University.

p. 106: In the acute phase of polio, when many children were placed in iron lungs to assist in respiration, every effort was made to comfort a sick child—photos from home and mementos made the separation slightly more bearable.

p. 107: Both parents of these two children were stricken by polio.

p. 109: A sister comforts her brother while he is still in need of assistance for respiration.

p. 112: On military bases, military aircraft and personnel were used to help transport polio patients.

p. 114: Physicians and a nurse in an acute care unit assist a patient wearing the protective garments used in managing all highly infectious diseases.

p. 115: Two brothers who contracted polio comfort each other in the hospital.

p. 117: In Hickory, North Carolina, the big epidemic of 1944 required the construction of a makeshift hospital in this rural town.

p. 118: This tiny baby is covered from her neck to her feet in hotpacks in an attempt to counteract the paralysis brought on by the polio virus.

p. 120: Temporary hospital in Hickory, North Carolina.

p. 121: This iron lung patient can read a book with a book holder attached to the top of the lung. What is not apparent from this photo, however, is the fact that frequently hurried medical staff could only come by once every hour or so and turn the page.

p. 123: This young polio patient is able to help herself get through her book by turning the pages with a page-turner using her mouth. Many inventions were developed to help paralyzed polio patients be more self-sufficient.

p. 124: This father-daughter duo contracted polio in 1953.

p. 125: The iron lung knew no age— children and adults of all ages with the most dreaded form of polio, bulbar polio, could find themselves captive to this respiration device.

p. 126: This young mother looks at a picture of her newborn child, delivered while she was in the iron lung.

p. 127: Hot pack therapy and massage were used to try to counter the crippling physical distortions caused by polio.

pp. 128 and 129: A sore backside was the result of the gamma globulin trials of 1953 which tried to stem the tide of polio outbreaks the summer before the Salk field trials.

p. 130: A warm water treatment was used to help rehabilitate the not-yet developed muscles of a baby who still needed to learn to walk.

p. 131: A father carries his daughter home from the hospital.

p. 132: A promotional picture of students looking over their "Polio Pointers" brochure during the 1954 field trials.

p. 133: The news aftermath of the April 12, 1955 announcement was universal and full of relief from the fear that had captured America for over half a century.

p. 136: When patients in iron lungs needed to be transported, the entire machine needed to be accommodated.

p. 137: This early iron lung would have been used in the 1930s and early 1940s.

p. 138: An iron lung ward for adults at Rancho Los Amigos.

p. 139: Breaking ground for the expansion of Rancho Los Amigos and those in wheelchairs give evidence as to why the expansion was necessary. (Courtesy of Rancho Los Amigos)

p. 140: Dr. John Affeldt, head of Rancho Los Amigos, during its expansion. (Courtesy of Rancho Los Amigos)

p. 141: Doctors and staff at the Rancho Los Amigos—one of the nation's foremost respiration centers sponsored by the March of Dimes in Southern California. (Courtesy of Rancho Los Amigos)

p. 142: When the upper body was affected by the disease, tasks such as eating a meal alone had to be totally relearned.

p. 143: Many March of Dimes photos picture a happy child in a difficult circumstance. But in reality, this child's life in the iron lung was difficult, tedious, and frequently frightening.

p. 144: Turning pages with a pointer allows a patient to be free of waiting for a nurse to turn a page.

p.145: The finished and newly modernized Rancho Los Amigos of the 1950s. (Courtesy of Rancho Los Amigos)

p. 148: A nurse stretches the leg muscles of a polio patient.

p. 149: This promotional photo taken by the March of Dimes gives the impression that nurses had time to read to polio patients and that, given the title of the book, that this child soon might go home and back to a normal child's life. Unfortunately, frequently neither of these images was true.

p. 150: This iron lung for an adult would have been used in the 1930s.

p. 151: A mother who contracted polio is surrounded by her three children who have come to visit her.

p. 152: This tiny baby, totally wrapped in hot packs, gets a cool drink from his juice bottle.

p. 154: This polio patient was chosen to appeal to the black population in the District of Columbia.

p. 155: Standing up again was difficult and this child shows the strain of doing what once, before polio, came naturally to him.

p. 158: Warm water baths sometimes helped to soothe paralyzed muscles of patients at Tuskegee.

p. 159: Every once in a while, children at Tuskegee, long separated from their parents, would be brought to a playground and take some respite from life on the ward.

p. 160: Making sure an unsteady child didn't hurt himself at Tuskegee, as well as at all polio facilities, was a high priority as children were pressed through the rehabilitation process.

p. 161: At Tuskegee, all of the patients were black, but it was also the only fully black-staffed facility in America—the doctors, the nurses, the physical therapists were all black. The bracemaker was the only white member of the Tuskegee team.

Chapter 5

pp. 162–163 background: Once the field trials were over, hundreds of thousands filed into school gymnasiums, public buildings, and medical centers across the nation to receive their three immunizations.

p. 163: The hundreds of culture tubes containing tissue which has been inoculated with virus and containing nutrient solution are placed in roller drums which turned slowly (about 10 to 12 revolutions in an hour) so that the tissue would be evenly bathed by the nutrient solution. Culture tubes are incubated for 7 to 8 days before being used for research and testing for the new vaccine.

p. 164: Davy Crockett's coonskin cap and the Salk shot became two symbols of the 1950s.

p. 165: During the epidemic in Hickory, North Carolina a small laboratory was established to test spinal fluids and blood samples from patients at the Emergency Infantile Paralysis Hospital.

p. 166: Dr. Albert Sabin shows his oral vaccine to a reporter during the field trials of 1960.

p. 167: The virus could not be seen until the advent of the electron microscope in 1938.

p. 168: Dr. Jonas Salk in his laboratory.

p. 169: Two scientists examine a model of the polio virus.

p. 170: Monkeys were at the center of polio research. For many years, it was only in live monkeys that the virus could be cultivated for scientific research. After the breakthrough discovery by Enders, Weller, and Robbins it only took one monkey kidney

to produce hundreds of portions of virus for testing.

p. 171: Dr. Jonas Salk administering his killed-virus vaccine during the field trials of 1954.

p. 172: Basil O'Connor and Dr. Jonas Salk—a duo that had the same obsession—the conquest of polio.

p. 173: Dr. Albert Sabin surveys an iron lung that he hopes will be made obsolete when the final results of his field trials are complete.

p. 174: Seven days after the announcement of the success of the field trials, this classroom gets ready to get their injections to prevent polio.

p. 175: Basil O'Connor (left) with Jonas Salk (center) and President Eisenhower (right). Eisenhower is presenting a commendation to Dr. Salk for the success of the field trials.

p. 177: Bottle of the newly tested polio vaccine.

p. 178: A poetic reminder that for polio victims, the vaccine was "too little, too late."

p. 180: Dr. Jonas Salk showing the experimental vaccine to CBS Correspondent Edward R. Murrow during the taping of a television broadcast intended to explain the complexities of the field trials to the American public.

p. 183: This little guy registers his disapproval of his participation in a field trial, in spite of his lollipop reward.

p. 185: The newspapers spread the good news about the success of the Salk vaccine.

p. 187: A total of the items used in the massive effort that was the 1954 Salk field trials.

p. 188: A telegram announces the release of the first lot of polio vaccine.

p. 192: At Armour Laboratories, gamma globulin was processed for the additional serum needed for the gamma globulin trials of 1953 and 1954.

p. 193: Maintaining a sufficient, healthy

monkey supply was critical to the success of the research and development phase of the vaccine.

p. 194: A technician at work in the laboratory.

p. 197: The "Polio Pioneer" promotional campaign featuring all of the children who received their trial vaccines and soon, hopefully, would never have to worry again about polio.

p. 201: Dr. Jonas Salk in his laboratory at the University of Pittsburgh

p. 202: When the vaccine was first introduced families would wait in long lines to be protected from polio.

p. 203: Children holding signs indicating the conventional wisdom of the days—myths or facts, no one knew, but all warnings from parents were repeated and heeded.

p. 204: Dr. Jonas Salk monitored every element of his laboratory, from the progress on lab results, to the correspondence of his secretary, to the construction of new rooms for the growing research teams.

p. 206: At the Institut de Neurologie Belge Research Laboratories scientists worked on polio research with a grant from the Rockefeller Foundation. The effort to find a vaccine went on throughout the Western World, led by the United States.

p. 209: Elvis Presley gets his polio shot in 1956 in an effort to promote immunization across America.

p. 213: Dr. Jonas Salk always seemed at once relaxed and obsessed by his commitment to finding the key to unlock polio.

p. 215: A gamma globulin production facility.

p. 217: After the 6- and 7-year-olds were inoculated the first year after the successful field trials, efforts were made to inoculate all Americans with the three shots necessary to provide immunity.

p. 220: Polio patients spent hours relearning tasks that once had come to them without a thought.

p. 224: Crowded hospital wards made it possible for children to develop friendships during what were frequently long hospital stays.

p. 228: Dr. Albert Sabin after the field trials of his live oral polio vaccine.

p. 229: Joseph Melnick holding a model of the virus that he intended to help conquer by use of the live virus vaccine.

Chapter 6

pp. 230–31 background: Polio patients congregate for a church service at Warm Springs.

p. 231: This polio poster by Milton Wynne was part of an exhibition sponsored by the Museum of Modern Art and the National Foundation for Infantile Paralysis in 1949.

p. 232: Social life at Warm Springs was critical in helping polios become comfortable living in an entirely new way.

p. 236: FDR didn't let his paralysis keep him from doing what he wanted. He enjoyed horseback riding at Warm Springs.

p. 239: Using parallel bars, polio patients were able to regain a sense of balance after having frequently been bedridden for many months.

p. 240: The brace shop at Warm Springs fitted each polio patient with exactly the right support for his or her body.

p. 242: Stretching in the warmth of the sunlight might make this painful exercise somewhat more bearable.

p. 247: A poster child teams up with Howdy Doody in the March of Dimes fundraising effort.

p. 248: On the ward, sometimes iron lungs could be positioned so patients could pass the time talking to each other.

p. 249: These adults are being trained to use their shoulders again in shoulder slings designed to build unparalyzed neck and arm muscles.

p. 251: People line up in a school gymnasium to receive the Sabin oral vaccine on sugar cubes.

p. 252: A mother reads to her daughter. Living in the iron lung was truly an "Alice in Wonderland"-like surrealistic experience.

p. 255: This is clearly a promotional picture with a happy child confined to an iron lung to be used in raising money for the March of Dimes.

p. 256: Muscle stretching was a daily part of rehabilitation that was quite painful, yet necessary, for a polio patient needing to keep paralyzing muscles from becoming atrophied.

p. 257: One of the many posters calling for assistance during the Mothers' March. These appeals played both to the public's fear of the disease and their sense of hope that something could be done about it if enough money could be raised.

p. 258: This promotional photograph is intended to demonstrate the activity of the March of Dimes in constructing the centers to house the waves of polio patients and rehabilitating the patients who came to them.

p. 259: This tiny baby is totally wrapped in hot packs.

p. 261: Sometimes elaborate mechanisms needed to be developed to encourage muscle development for even the simplest tasks.

p. 262: A polio patient learns to feed himself with his toes.

p. 263: Protection came too late for this wheelchair-bound polio survivor.

p. 265: No longer able to mend her children's clothes by hand, this mother learns to manipulate a sewing machine and the arm slings to mend her children's clothes.

p. 266: In arm slings and hand braces, this young polio patient learns to type.

p. 269: The entire family, with the assistance of a public health nurse, was always called upon to care for a family member brought home in the iron lung.

p. 270: Taking the first steps at Tuskegee.

p. 271: A hand brace makes written communication possible again.

p. 272: Strengthening exercise class for polio patients was a part of daily life before leaving the hospital.

p. 273: This respirator patient, Irene Ridgeway, became famous for her paintings rendered through a paintbrush held in her mouth.

Afterword

pp. 274–275 background: A line of Ethiopians wait for polio vaccination. (Courtesy of Rotary International)

p. 275: Polio continues as a crippler in much of the Third World. India has been the hardest hit. (Courtesy of Rotary International)

p. 276: A young Kenyan polio survivor with his crutches and leg braces. (Courtesy of Rotary International)

p. 277: The children remain polio's saddest victims. (Courtesy of Rotary International)

p. 278: In spite of its eradication in the Western Hemisphere polio is still a danger to the impoverished families of the Third World. (Courtesy of Rotary International)

p. 279: Vaccination programs bring protection to this Ethiopian baby on National Immunization Day. (Courtesy of Rotary International)

p. 280, top: This young Indian boy has the withered legs of a polio survivor. (Courtesy of Rotary International)

p. 280, bottom: A young Indian mother holds her child for vaccination. (Courtesy of Rotary International)